The Great Dental Deception
EXPOSED

The mercury based dental amalgam was introduced to the United States in 1833. Its usage over the past 170 years is the cause of illness, disease and death. Mercury is the most toxic non-radioactive element on our planet. Dentists stuff this element into dental cavities; the mercury vapor is inhaled 24 hours per day and accumulates in every cell and every organ in the human body. This creates illness. A plethora of scientific research proves mercury amalgams are very dangerous, yet the American Dental Association (ADA) endorses its usage in infants, children, pregnant moms, elderly people, as well as you and me.

If you broke a mercury-based thermometer would you willingly breathe the mercury vapor? The answer is of course no, but it is analogous to current dental procedures. Your dental filling is the same vapor.

When the truth surfaces, the resultant lawsuits against everyone remotely associated with the dental profession will be enormous. The magnitude of the damages will make the tobacco settlements look like petty cash.

ANNE HERFF MEYER, DDS, LLC
SEA TOWNE - NORTH COURTYARD
1660 N. COAST HIGHWAY
NEWPORT, OR 97365-2357

PREFACE

THE GREAT DENTAL DECEPTION is authored by a patient who is and will continue to recover from the effects of mercury being released from dental fillings.

The book is based on the simple fact that mercury, the second most toxic substance on our planet, is used in dental fillings. The dental industry is aware that mercury is released from our fillings and poisons us. But the American Dental Association (ADA), the American Medical Association (AMA) and other government regulatory agencies refuse to alert us to the dangers. In fact our policies actually conceal the science behind the dangers of mercury in our dental fillings. When "activists" attempt to implement informed consent as it relates to mercury amalgams, the ADA argues against informing consumers that dental fillings even contain mercury. They do not want the public made aware that a toxic substance is used in mouths. The simple questions is – why the cover-up?

The reference to thermometers is because it is the most commonly known product containing mercury. Mercury is used in many thermometers as a way of determining temperature. Fortunately, advanced technologies are in the process of making the traditional mercury thermometer obsolete. In fact many retailers now refuse to stock mercury based thermometers because of their dangers. In addition, a Congressional bill proposes to eliminate all thermometers that contain mercury. Nevertheless, if you look around you can find a mercury-based thermometer; break one open and inhale the vapors. It causes illness quicker than dental fillings, but it is the same type of poison.

Once the truth is uncovered about current dental procedures the litigation that will take place will be record breaking. Malpractice lawsuits against the dental industry will spare no one.

The goal of this book is to educate the reader regarding information that is currently available on mercury dental amalgams. The hope is that you will accept the information presented, and make decisions that help restore your health, insure your quality of life in the future, and help make well thought out decisions for family members. Health is really a choice between two different concepts: medication or education. If you chose medication, doctors write prescriptions and dictate not only your quality of life, but also ultimately how long you will live. If you opt for education, you become a knowledgeable consumer of healthcare options and make decisions that improve your quality of life. You are in charge of your health; it is not delegated to others.

There is a great deal of information available regarding mercury amalgams; however, the search for information can be laborious, especially for someone who is sick. My hope is this book provides the most current research and information so it's easy to become knowledgeable. The book has intentionally omitted an index – the hope is that the reader will read the book from cover to cover. There is a danger in providing an index thus providing a link to a specific subject. Everything related to mercury toxicity is connected, and therefore understanding the entire process is critical for recovery.

In order to understand the information presented you must have an open mind or be blessed with the desire to become smarter than you were before you read this book. If you feel traditional medicine is correct 100% of the time, you made a mistake purchasing this book. However, if you believe medicine and health are still evolving this book will prove, to anyone that reads it, that current dental procedures are dangerous and life threatening.

Webster's definition of wisdom states, *"The power of true and right discernment, using sound judgment, common sense, a high degree of knowledge."* All of us are blessed with the opportunity to gain wisdom and utilize it. Most of us have displayed these traits in our various careers, our family life, or in our education.

Being wise or displaying wisdom is not defined as conforming to conventional doctrine. While you read this book, you should begin to understand the horrific dangers of mercury amalgams, and then make a choice: either get in the uneducated parade and go along with traditional thinking and ignore the scientific facts relating to mercury amalgams, or use sound judgment and common sense based on your increased knowledge of the subject. If you do the latter, you will join the growing ranks of wise people who object to the current use of mercury amalgams. If you chose to have your mercury amalgams replaced, the odds are you will enjoy both a better quality of life and a longer life.

A portion of the proceeds of this book will be donated to Dental Amalgam Syndrome (DAMS), and Consumers for Dental Choice. These are non-profit organizations that educate consumers on the dangers of mercury-filled dental amalgams. It is my opinion the best way to change current thinking is to educate the consumer. Our politicians are inept in spite of studies that prove mercury amalgams are dangerous, our regulatory agencies, the Food and Drug Administration (FDA), Centers for Disease Control and Prevention (CDC), and Environmental Protection Agency (EPA) are seemingly clueless or simply uninterested, the ADA, AMA and other trade organizations try to confuse the issue with an historical perspective versus science, and insurance companies seem interested in addressing symptoms, not cures. Thus, it is up to the consumer to change things. Books, news articles, and web sites help and organizations like DAMS and Consumers for Dental Choice can make a difference.

I sincerely hope the information in this book helps you attain a healthier and happy life. God speed.

A DEBT OF GRATITUDE

This book is dedicated to the passionate research accomplished over the past 100 years that proves the dangers of mercury amalgams. The individuals that deserve accolades are Pinto, Price, Vimy, Huggins, Stock, Haley, Ziff, and many others that I am sure that I have failed to mention. These pioneers have and continue to change the way dentistry is practiced in the 21st century.

Recently a number of political and legal activists, including DAMS and Consumers for Dental Choice, have altered the traditional authority exercised by dental boards and lawsuits are being filed with great frequency. Change is forthcoming.

In addition to the above individuals, each day numerous dentists abandon the use of mercury amalgams for biocompatible non-toxic materials. Their courage should be praised since the American Dental Association and state dental boards harass many of these dentists and in some cases threaten their license. Without a license these dentists can no longer remove mercury from a patient's mouth, which is so important in order for many people to regain their health.

Finally, accolades to countries that have limited the use of mercury amalgams. The research and science that caused these countries to pass laws changing how mercury amalgams are used provides a better quality of life for their population.

From a personal viewpoint;
Brian the book would never have been completed without your help
Sandy without your initial proof read this would have been jibberish
Maria-Elaina thanks for the title idea, and final thoughts
Craig thanks for all the computer assistance

ISBN #0-9749869-0-9

Library of Congress Catalog Card Number 2004101681

INTRODUCTION

Recently I was having a discussion with a group of friends and we all began by speculating what we would do if we hit the lottery. Since I have some investment experience, I was asked what I would recommend doing with a large sum of money. I pondered this question for only a few seconds. And I am sure everyone thought I would suggest using some of it to buy a second home, a boat or even a country club membership. The rest of it could certainly be invested in a variety of stocks and bonds. I am sure this would be the conclusion that 99.9% of people would advise. After contemplating the obvious, my recommendation was that the best, the very best use of this money and the number one priority would be to have every member of their family go to the dentist and have their mercury amalgams removed. This simple process would add years to their life allowing them to earn even more money, and most importantly, have plenty of extra years of life to enjoy the luck that the lottery brought them. After removing this poison from their bodies, then look at buying that second home or invest in that great stock opportunity.

I am sure some people reading this wonder why I made such a strange suggestion. The answer to this is obvious to some of us – those of us poisoned by our mercury amalgams. The answer to others is baffling since most people have never heard about this medical malady unless they read certain homeopathic or alternative medicine books or books like this written by individuals who understand mercury poisoning based on personal experience. Why does your doctor or dentist not tell you about this? Why is it that many countries in Europe have limited mercury amalgams, but in our country of medical breakthroughs we are oblivious to the problem? Why is it that there are numerous stories of people regaining their health by having mercury removed from their teeth but no one in mainstream medicine wants to address it? I cannot answer these questions. I can tell you, however, that mercury amalgams make people extremely sick, and they will kill people. To put it rather succinctly: if you have mercury in your mouth, you should have it removed.

This book provides information for individuals who are mercury toxic and want to regain their health. It also provides information for people who simply want to insure themselves better long-term health by having their mercury amalgams removed. If a reader does not have mercury amalgams, I doubt they will ever let a dentist place them in their mouth. There are many books and newsletters available, but few of these are authored or written by a patient. I was in poor health for many years, and I went the traditional route for solutions before I turned to alternatives and learned the source of my poor health was mercury poisoning. I tried many things in order to detoxify, and hopefully some of my real life experiences will help others heal faster.

One other thing to note is that research is taking place daily on this subject. Most of the new information is coming from Europe, so in addition to reading this book, keep appraised of research that is making detoxification easier and faster.

The following web sites are worthwhile:
www.toxicteeth.com
www.iaomt.com
www.altcorp.com
www.vimy-dentistry.com
www.vaccinessafey.edu/thi-table.htm
www.bioprobe.com
www.hugnet.com
www.amalgam.org
www.holistic.com/dental/amalgam
www.mercuryfilling.com
www.home.earthlink.net/~berniew/
www.cavitat.com
www.CFSN.com
www.healthydetox.org
www.mercola.com
www.dentistry-toothtruth.com
www.authismresearchinstitute.com
www.nueroreport.com
www.atsdr.cdc.gov/toxfaq.html
www.vaccinationnews.com

New sites are constantly being added thus it is worthwhile to search "mercury fillings."

Dr. Weston Price once stated, *"A new truth can come only to a properly prepared mind."* The scientific research that is available supports the truth that mercury amalgams are dangerous. The mind has been prepared; it is time for the truth to be accepted.

TABLE OF CONTENTS

CHAPTER 1

For The Lord Gives Wisdom And From His Mouth Comes Knowledge And Understanding

TRUE FALSE TEST

To make the test easier, the answers will be given in advance. **The following statements are all true.** These facts will provide insight and understanding as to the enormous dangers of mercury generally, and mercury amalgam fillings specifically.

1. Mercury is the most toxic non-radioactive substance in the universe.
2. Mercury is the second most toxic substance in the universe – second only to plutonium.
3. The World Health Organization has determined that mercury fillings are the primary source of human mercury contamination.
4. The EPA has issued a mandate that mercury amalgams that are not used in your teeth are dangerous materials. According to EPA guidelines, it is a felony to buy them in the ground or not dispose of them appropriately.
5. Phiny in the 1st century B.C., described illness in slaves who worked in mercury mines.
6. Aristotle called mercury "living silver" or "quicksilver" because of its volatility to any stimulus.
7. Mercury was first introduced, as a medicinal product, in the 16th century by the German physician Paracelsus. The fact that mercury changed the color of a person's stool from brown to green suggested to the medical community that bad bile was being eliminated. Thus, mercury became an appropriate metal for anyone with an illness to ingest. In reality, mercury was damaging the good bacteria in the intestinal track that keeps the pigment of stools brown. Nevertheless, mercury was used extensively for many decades for a variety of maladies.
8. Multiple Sclerosis (MS) patients have eight times higher levels of mercury in their cerebrospinal fluid when compared to neurologically healthy individuals.

9.   Inorganic mercury is capable of producing symptoms that are indistinguishable from those of MS. Some people diagnosed with MS are actually mercury poisoned.

10.   Recent autopsy studies in Europe show a correlation between the number of dental amalgams and mercury levels in the brain and kidney.

11.   Dr. David Eggleson of the University of California found a T lymphocyte count of 47% (norm 80%) in patients with mercury fillings. After removal of the patient's mercury fillings, the T lymphocyte count rose to 73%.

12.   Mercury is used as a preservative in vaccines, flu shots and allergy shots. The preservative is called Thimesosal. The mercury kills any bacteria that might exist in the vaccine. In addition studies demonstrate that the mercury in vaccines is absorbed into cells and thus organs.

13.   Four people died of mercury poisoning in Michigan in 1989. What was the cause of their deaths? One of the four people had been heating amalgams in an effort to remove the silver. Not only did the mercury vapor kill the four people who lived in the house, but the house also had to be destroyed because it could not be decontaminated.

14.   In 1957 in a thermometer factory in Brooklyn, three people died because the company used dangerous procedures when dealing with mercury. OSHA was aware of the problems and tried to get compliance. After the deaths, the owners faced criminal indictments.

15.   A "quack" is defined as someone who pretends to cure a problem. In the 1800's, people who used mercury to cure illnesses were referred to as quacks. (From the German word for quicksilver; quack silver)

16.   Mercury was the god of commerce in the Roman Empire. This god was associated with trickery, stealing and slight of hand.

17.   The term "mad as a hatter" did not originate with Alice in Wonderland or the mad hatter tea party. In the 1800s, the hat industry used a combination of mercury and nitric acid to make felt hats. The workers/hatters breathed the mercury vapors all day and the vapors caused numerous neurological symptoms leading to the phrase "mad as a hatter."

18.   The first reported case of MS was in 1838. Parkinson's Disease was described in 1817 by Dr Parkinson.

19. Studies indicate individuals without amalgams have lower blood pressure than people with mercury amalgams.
20. 85% of all Americans have at least one mercury amalgam.
21. Dentists use 100 tons of mercury every year. The vast majority believes it is harmless in your mouth.
22. In 1989 the EPA declared amalgams a hazardous substance and they must be disposed of under strict guidelines.
23. In 1990 *60 Minutes* aired a devastating exposé on amalgams.
24. In 1990 the EPA banned mercury in paint.
25. George Washington died either from a common cold or mercury poisoning. Washington had cold symptoms and his doctor bled him (common practice in the 1700s), and provided him with a dose of mercury. His doctor repeated the process the next day. The following day he died.
26. President Andrew Jackson died of heavy metal poisoning. The Armed Forces Institute of Pathology did two comprehensive laboratory analyses on Jackson's hair. In 1815 he had a mercury level of 6.0 with a normal range of 1-1.2. In 1839 his mercury level was 5.8. They also did a lead test and his level in 1815 was 130 with a normal range 0-20, and in 1839 it had decreased to 69. The reason for the drop in lead was that 2 lead bullets were removed. The mercury level and both lead levels are considered extraordinarily high.
27. Meriwether Lewis committed suicide after completing his infamous expedition to the Pacific Northwest. It is thought that he suffered from depression after an incredible journey and thus took his own life. It is also known that his entire expedition contracted syphilis numerous times from Native Americans. The treatment for syphilis at this time was mercury. Depression is a common symptom of mercury poisoning.
28. According to OSHA, mercury is a poison at microscopic levels; any inhalation is extremely dangerous.
29. Mercury adversely affects the heart, liver, brain, kidneys and other organs.
30. In 1993, German amalgam manufacturer, De Gussa, discontinued its production of mercury amalgams out of fear of lawsuits.
31. OSHA, the government agency that insures safe working conditions, uses a meter to measure mercury in the workplace. If the reading is above 20 micrograms per cubic meter, the company is fined and closed until levels are within the proper range. All employees in such a situation are monitored for mercury toxicity.

A mouth full of amalgams can have a reading of 50-150 micrograms. Mouths with multiple amalgams do not pass OSHA requirements.

32. The average amalgam filling weighs one gram. The mercury portion is .5 grams. The average American has 10 amalgams or 5 grams of mercury in their mouth.

33. 0.5 grams of mercury in a 10-acre lake would result in the EPA issuing a warning and an advisory not to eat fish in the lake. The mercury content of the fish would be dangerous to your health.

34. 225 million Americans have mercury amalgam fillings.

35. U. S. government studies document that 100% of Americans have detectable levels of toxic chemicals or heavy metals.

36. Autoimmune diseases are increasing at an alarming rate and being diagnosed at younger and younger ages.

37. Only 10% of Americans are aware that their dental amalgams contain mercury.

38. Over 60,000 people from all over the world have overcome a variety of illnesses and health problems when their mercury amalgams were removed.

These studies, statements, and anecdotal stories describe the problems mercury poses for everyone. They also demonstrate the challenge our immune system has in keeping us healthy. It's fair to state that in order to battle many of the 21st century diseases, it's critical to have a healthy immune system. It is possible to have a healthy immune system if you have mercury amalgams.

Thomas Edison stated: *"The doctor of the future will give no medicine but will interest his patients in the care of the human frame, in diet and in the cause and prevention of disease."*

As you read the following chapters, it will become apparent to you that one of the causes of disease is the mercury vapor in mercury amalgams.

CHAPTER 2

Blessed is the man who finds wisdom

ABE LINCOLN WITH MERCURY AND PRESIDENT LINCOLN WITHOUT MERCURY

President Lincoln is well known for the Emancipation Proclamation and standing firm in the face of Civil War. Most Americans consider him our greatest President. However, Lincoln is often described by historians as moody, depressed, quick-tempered, with drawn and often times forgetful. Most of these personality descriptions are accurate, particularly before he became President of the United States. Lincoln was prescribed a medication called "blue mass" and in the 19th century, this pill was used to cure a number of maladies including "melancholy," irritability and absent-mindedness. "Blue mass" was a mercury-based medication. Mercury was a common prescription in our history and various forms of mercury were used for many either real or perceived illnesses.

An extract from author William Herndon describes Lincoln: "He would without warning burst out in a loud laugh or quickly spring up and run downstairs as if his house was on fire without saying anything." A colleague, Henry Clay Whitney, wrote he awoke one morning and saw his friend Lincoln "talking the wildest and most incoherent nonsense all to himself." He also described period of "majestic and terrifying wrath." During this period, Lincoln was taking "blue mass". President Lincoln determined "blue mass made him cross" and he stopped taking it five months after his election as president. Subsequently, John Nicolay, Lincoln's secretary, wrote, "Under the most trying conditions and circumstances, and during the whole time, I never saw him manifest any extraordinary excitement . . . or indulge in any violence of speech or action beyond that of impressive emphasis."

It seems Lincoln attributed his personality disorder to taking "blue mass". He stopped taking it and led his country through one of its most trying periods: the Civil War and the beginnings of Reconstruction. If he had

5

continued taking mercury compounds and assumed the role as a mad hatter, one can only speculate how our society would be different.

Researchers at the University of Minnesota attempted to replicate "blue mass". They followed the 19th century formula using elemental mercury (basically the same type of mercury that is a component of amalgams), with the herbs that were also incorporated at that time. The pill was then sent to a laboratory for analysis. The process used a mercury vapor analysis and then replicated the digestion and ultimate absorption into the bloodstream. Assuming two to three pills were taken daily the lab concluded that 130-185 mgs of mercury was ingested each day, *which is 9000 times above today's acceptable levels.* In his early days, many labeled Lincoln as "nuts." If he was, then it is clear the mercury compounds he was taking were to blame. Fortunately he decided to stop poisoning himself and his self-diagnosis changed our country forever.

WE LIVE IN A TOXIC WORLD

Think about our world today versus 20 years ago, 50 years ago and 100 years ago. First, our food is not as nutritious as it was in the past. Today we eat highly processed foods and our intake of fast foods from restaurants dominates many lives. In addition, most doctors state very few people get enough fiber. Simply put, we are not nourished by our food like we were in the past. Since our fiber intake is low, we retain various toxins in our body for a much longer period of time. If these toxins are not eliminated through bowel movements, the toxins are absorbed by various tissues and cells within our body, and ultimately cause chronic illness, and eventually, disease. Naturopathic physicians and many physicians in Europe believe everyone should have three bowel movements per day. How many people pass that test? Good diet and appropriate transit time in the intestines are absolutely critical for good heath.

It is interesting what happens to cultures that are "civilized." Prior to the 1940's, Eskimos in Northern Canada had no exposure to western culture. As this group began eating the "new" diet women began to develop breast cancer, teenagers developed acne, and maladies such as diabetes, heart disease, high blood pressure and obesity all became commonplace. Prior to 1940 these maladies were all unheard of in the Eskimo villages of North Canada.

An interesting study took place in the Pacific Islands in which three islands were studied. People living on Pukapuka averaged about 1800 calories per day, which included about 70 grams of fat and 9 grams of sugar, mostly from fruit. Their diet was traditional island culture. People on the island of Rarotonga had a diet of both traditional island food and western food. Their average calorie intake was about 2100, with 63 grams of fat and 35 grams of sugar. The Maori of New Zealand eat a totally modern diet, 2500 calories, 125 grams of fat per day, and 71 grams of sugar per day. The average American consumes 125 grams of sugar per day.

On Rarotonga, gross obesity is 5.2 times greater than Pukapuka; on Maori, obesity is 13 times greater than Pukapuka. Diabetes is 6 times greater for the Maori than on Pukapuka. Heart disease is 2 times higher on Rarotonga and Maori than on Pukapuka. And both the Maori and the Rarotonga, high blood pressure is seen in 10 times more people than on Pukapuka.

Today's diet has shifted our priorities as it relates to disease. Today one in three of us will die of cancer, 1 in 3 has allergies and 1 in 5 suffers from some sort of mental illness. Heart disease represents 40% of all deaths and 1 in 5 pregnancies ends in a miscarriage. This represents a dramatic change in the lat 100 years. To most this is a disturbing trend.

The marketing of the western diet in magazines and on television commercials is both guaranteeing disease and an earlier death. Nevertheless, we have bought the television commercials, not the research. Drug companies prosper from a "civilized" diet since they can sell drugs that treat the symptoms of today's diet. We need to change our eating habits in order to increase in our quality and duration of life.

We now deal with a host of toxins that are readily recognized by mainstream medicine, which include fuel exhaust, industrial waste, and a plethora of pesticides, fungicides, radiation, compromised drinking water, environmental pollution, and cigarette smoke. Add to this list the damage heavy metals, especially mercury, lead and aluminum are doing to our bodies and it is amazing that anyone is healthy today. The obvious conclusion is that we all could be healthier with changes in not only our life style, but also in our nutrition as well.

Our environment is poisoning our bodies; add to that we do not get anywhere close to the proper nutrients from our food, and it is not surprising so many people are sick. The simple solution is that we can either move to an environmentally safe place, for instance, the wilderness where we can grow organic food and breathe clean air, or we can support our bodies with the proper food, and necessary supplements to combat the above toxins. Later in this book we will discuss supplements that will help battle this war on toxins. You cannot protect yourself from an unhealthy environment without supplements, and the dosages of these necessary supplements are much greater than the RDA's you read about in various books. To win the war on toxins, including mercury poisoning, you must take the proper vitamins, minerals and herbs. Proper supplementation will enhance our metabolic functions and provide the extra ingredients you need for your quality of life. In addition to supplements, it is important to eat untreated foods, raw foods, and drink fresh juices. Finally as much as possible, eat organic food.

THE MERCURY-BASED THERMOMETER

Before we discuss dental fillings that contain mercury here are a few comments on the traditional thermometer.

The mercury thermometer has existed for decades. It contains about .75 grams of mercury that is encased in glass. As long as it remains enclosed, there are no problems. However, when released, in case the glass is broken or punctured, it poses a serious health challenge, potentially more disastrous than cancer or heart disease. Fortunately, after years of use it is being replaced by 21st century technology that can determine temperature without using toxic substances.

Here are a few tragic stories from the Environmental Protection Agency (EPA) regarding the traditional mercury based thermometer:

1. Two people died when a broken thermometer was placed in a pan on a heated stove. The vapor was easily inhaled causing death from mercury poisoning.
2. A small child was hospitalized after inhaling mercury vapor from a broken thermometer. When the thermometer broke some of the mercury seeped into the carpet. Although everyone thought the problem was properly handled, the child inhaled a small amount of vapor while playing on the carpet.
3. Three children ages 18 months to 6 years old were hospitalized after inhaling mercury vapor from a thermometer that broke and spilled onto the living room carpet.

The EPA has made a few comments regarding the health risks of mercury:

1. Swallowed mercury is not dangerous. It passes through the GI tract without being absorbed. It is mercury vapor that poses the serious problem.
2. If mercury is spilled do not vacuum it. The heat and rapid air circulation causes mercury to vaporize. Mercury is very volatile.
3. The EPA claims symptoms of mercury poisoning from a broken thermometer include the following: tremors, vision and or hearing changes, insomnia, difficulty with memory, headaches, irritability, shyness, nervousness, rashes, itching, joint pain, and excessive sweating. These are some of the same symptoms that appear in mercury poisoning from inhaling vapors from mercury amalgams. It makes sense because mercury poisoning, regardless of the source, should exhibit the same symptoms.

The EPA makes the following recommendations on what actions to take if you break a thermometer while using it:

1. Ventilate the room. Close off the room from the rest of the house. Try and isolate the mercury to one room.
2. Pick up the mercury beads with an index card. Do not break the beads into additional beads; these will more easily disperse into other areas.
3. Don't use any type of household cleaner. Ammonia and chlorine will react with mercury causing the release of a toxic gas.
4. Once the beads are collected, put them into a zip lock bag. Put the zip lock bag into a second zip lock bag, put the second zip lock bag into a third zip lock bag. Then put the three bags into a plastic container that is also sealed. Immediately take this to the closest hazardous waste disposal site. Call the EPA.

The EPA suggests that people should use a great deal of caution when mercury spills from a thermometer. The mercury vapor that can be created is clearly very dangerous. Did you know that every dental amalgam in your mouth creates the same vapor that the EPA warns against?

WHAT COMPRISES A DENTAL FILLING?

Many of us go to the dentist every six months for a dental check up. Periodically we are informed that we have a cavity. The dentist then "numbs" the area around the tooth with the cavity and we obtain a filling. That is the most any of us know, including unfortunately, the dentist. In the filling is a concoction of metals that, when mixed together, harden in our tooth to provide a dental surface. The filling we receive is called a mercury amalgam.

The definition of mercury amalgam is the union of mercury with another metal. In all probability you remember the dentist or the hygienist mixing this product on a table next to the dental chair. The mixture is a combination of mercury, silver, copper, tin, nickel and possibly other trace metals. Mercury compromises 50-70% of the final product, with copper typically representing the 2nd highest portion. There are many different combinations, but generally these are the components inserted into your tooth. Most of us assumed this was a safe restoration since the pain disappeared and we seemingly had no side effects from the dental procedure. But were we ever wrong. A simple mercury amalgam with a surface area of only 0.5 square centimeters will release 15 micrograms of mercury per day. To understand this completely, if a filling contains 50% mercury when it was placed in our mouth, when it falls out naturally only 15% remains. The other 35% was distributed to our kidneys, liver, heart, brain etc. The dentist inserted a poison in our mouth that will be inhaled and absorbed through our lungs into every organ in our body. For many people the mercury amalgam causes disease and death.

MERCURY AS PART OF THE DENTAL AMALGAM

The simple question that must be answered is *What are the toxic effects of mercury and the impact that results from mercury in the dental amalgam?* Previous sections suggest that mercury is highly toxic and dentists should no longer use it. But prior to drawing that conclusion let's address the question presented. The answer will be presented in two fashions. The obvious presentation is from science. In other words, learning about mercury from a scientific viewpoint can help answer the basic question, *Is mercury in your dental filling dangerous?* The other is to hear about patient histories in order to glean an understanding about mercury and the effects it can have on men, women and even children.

Mercury is a heavy silvery metallic element. Its symbol is Hg and it is number 80 on the periodic table. The unique property of mercury is that mercury is a liquid at room temperature; it is very unstable, and extremely volatile.

Mercury can take many forms. The most common form of mercury is metallic mercury (Hg*). Metallic mercury, or elemental mercury, creates mercury vapor, which is both colorless and odorless. Mercury amalgams contain 50% metallic mercury. Mercury vapor is created when metallic mercury vaporizes. Mercury vapor is lipid soluble and thus readily passes through cell membranes and across the blood brain barrier.

Mercury vapor has access to every cell and tissue; through a metabolic process it is oxidized to Hg++. This new form of mercury is far more toxic than Hg* since it is not easily removed from cells. When Hg++ combines with carbon it transforms to organic mercury. Methyl mercury (MeHg) is the most common form of organic mercury. It is absorbed easily, passes thru the blood brain barrier and causes changes in the DNA structure of cells.

Through the simple act of chewing, mercury vapor is released from the mercury amalgam; it is inhaled and within 15 minutes absorbed into your bloodstream. Research proves that almost 100% of the mercury vapor that is created by a mercury amalgam is inhaled and absorbed. Mercury vapor then passes through cell membranes and crosses the blood brain barrier. Mercury has access to every organ in your body. Mercury vapor has the ability to transform to every type of mercury mentioned through the natural metabolic processes in the human body. Through the simple process of chewing you create every toxic type of mercury described above.

From our brief chemistry lesson we know that mercury is a deadly element. Remember, it has been proven that mercury is released from our fillings and when released from our fillings it is inhaled via our lungs and distributed to various organs. The simple fact is that all the various forms of mercury are toxic, and when absorbed replaces zinc, magnesium, and other critical minerals at various binding sites in our body. The result of this action causes illness, disease and ultimately death.

THE HISTORY OF DENTISTRY IN THE UNITED STATES

In the late 1700's and early 1800's there were two types of dentists in the United States. The first was the traditional medical doctor who also tended to his patient's dental needs. The second was anyone who wanted to be a dentist. This group was typically comprised of barbers, woodworkers, blacksmiths and other trades that practiced dentistry in its crudest form. Anyone that wanted to be a dentist could become one simply by hanging a sign in their window advertising dentistry. At this time there was no anesthesia, and tooth extractions were the common solution. Early writings of dentists describe the painful process that all patients encountered 200 years ago.

In 1833 the Crawcour brothers introduced the mercury amalgam into this country. An advertising blitz by the Crawcour's created the opportunity for these two con men to dupe the public. They had a great deal of success in Europe with their mercury amalgam process and when they came to the United States with their product there were no regulating agencies to analyze their mixture. They simply sold its virtues.

Until then a patient in pain had two options: one was to have the tooth pulled and second, somewhat rare, was to have gold pounded into the cavity area. With the introduction of ROYAL MINERAL SUCCEDANEUM (this is the name the Crawcours used in advertising the mercury amalgam) a patient could have the discomfort solved in only minutes. In 1833 the dentist that used this new mixture simply molded it around the cavity without first drilling out the decay. The patient received a painless solution; therefore it had to be better than any of the prior methods. No mention was ever made in the advertising that mercury was used in the product. Since this was quick and easy most dentists adopted its usage. A few of the more qualified dentists objected to its usage and specifically, usage of mercury. But ease and practicality prevailed 170 years ago. Remember the primary dentists of that time were uneducated craftsmen. Many probably had no idea what they were putting into people's mouths and even if they knew that mercury was the primary product, most would not have known that the consequences were deadly.

The medical doctors of that time understood the serious problems mercury could cause, and they immediately created the first dental school in order to try and bring order from this chaos. And the medical doctors in New York also formed the first dental society in order to protect the public from inappropriate care. One outcome of this new society was that the Crawcour's were kicked out of the country.

With the creation of the first dental school and the first professional association, dentistry was on the road toward becoming a science and not an occupation of quacks. In 1840 this trend continued when a national association of dentists was formed: The American Society of Dental Surgeons. In 1843 this organization banned the use of the mercury amalgam. It was unsafe for the public to use. However, many dentists and patients still wanted to use the mercury amalgam because it was easy, inexpensive, and fast. And not unlike today, education regarding the product was either ignored or not well understood. Based on the pressure the society was getting, it rescinded its ban in 1850 in hopes of rekindling membership. But at this point the society was doomed and it finally disbanded in 1856.

In 1859 amalgam dentists formed a new organization. It was called the American Dental Association, also known to some as the **Amalgam Death Association.** This association was comprised of dentists whose only concern was filling a tooth quickly, easily and inexpensively. No research was done on the product put in the tooth or the effect it had on other parts of the human body. Furthermore, dental schools educated dentists on only the teeth and the mouth. But since dental schools were nothing more than trade schools, the education probably would have not mattered. It was not until the early 1900's that a high school diploma was necessary to enter a dental school. In retrospect, the birth of the ADA was the result of the desire of uneducated craftsmen to use mercury amalgams.

The ADA is 143 years old and continues to defend the use of mercury amalgams. Regardless of the fact that research continues to prove that mercury amalgams cause illness, the ADA steadfastly states it is a safe dental material. This stance is becoming more and more difficult for the ADA to defend.

Dr. Carl Svare of the University of Iowa proved that mercury vapors are released from mercury based amalgams. Because of this, the ADA admitted that mercury amalgams release mercury. Dr. Svare had patients with mercury amalgams and without mercury amalgams chew gum for 10 minutes. He then measured their breath when they exhaled. Those patients with mercury amalgams had a 15-fold increase in mercury vapor after chewing gum and those without mercury amalgams had the same base number as they had prior to chewing gum. Thus the ADA had to affirm that some mercury is released from dental fillings when a person simply chews. And most of it is inhaled through your lungs and distributed to various organs. The ADA claims most of the mercury is eliminated in urine. This is simply not true. Some is eliminated in urine, but most mercury exits the body via the feces. The truth is that most is absorbed and deposited in vital organs. It is important to remember mercury is the most toxic non-radioactive element in our universe.

Conclusion: You are inhaling a deadly poison every time you breathe even if you only have one mercury amalgam.

Following the University of Iowa study, the ADA released information to its constituents (the dentist, not the patient), suggesting safety measures to adhere to when using mercury. The following are some of the measures that dentists must use when using mercury in their practice:

. . **"There must be a fresh air exchange, i.e. good ventilation, in the dental office in order to allow mercury to be exchanged for clean air (oxygen)."**

This criterion certainly assists the dentist, the staff and the patient while in the office, but I wonder how the human body can be ventilated in order to exchange mercury for oxygen? We do not have very good windows or other ways to exchange mercury for healthy elements. Thus, the mercury must be trapped in our body, and this will be proved as you continue reading future sections of this book. According to the ADA, this is not a problem.

. . **"Do not have carpeting in the dental office, it absorbs mercury and makes decontamination difficult."**

If a specialist cannot remove mercury out of a carpet, I wonder how a human body with livers, a heart, and a brain can purify itself from this deadly poison.

. . **"Mercury must be stored in an unbreakable container and kept away from heat. Heat increases the rate mercury vapor is released. It should be stored at room temperature."**

14

We already know that mercury leaches from our fillings, and that we have a body temperature of 98.6 degrees. We store mercury in a tooth at a temperature well above ADA guidelines.

. . "When removing amalgams dentists should have a filter that traps the amalgam, and any scraps should be stored in a tightly closed container."

This is good advice for the dentist. But when mercury is put in our mouth our only filters are the liver, kidney, and skin. This certainly proves why these particular organs are severely compromised when a person has multiple mercury amalgams in their mouth. This is discussed in greater detail later in the book.

. . "Do not touch or handle mercury amalgams."

The ADA is telling the dentist they should not touch or handle mercury without gloves. So why is it OK to put this in a patient's mouth? This logic is absurd. Dentists cannot touch the mercury amalgam mixture without gloves on. However, It is okay to stuff as much of this poison as necessary into a person's mouth.

It seems we have a serious paradox. These are guidelines that attempt to spare dentists the harm and the toxic effects of mercury, but there are no guidelines for the patient. With just a little intuitive thinking, it is clear that putting mercury in our mouth is dangerous.

The ADA did address the consumer when it published a brochure: "Answers to Your Questions About Silver Fillings." The marketing brochure makes a number of statements that are false and deceptive.

First the title of the brochure is misleading because mercury amalgams are not silver fillings. *Silver is used in the amalgam, but it represents an inconsequential percent of the mixture.* They are mercury fillings and all literature should reflect the truth. Since the ADA has a "gag order" on dentists in every state except Oregon and Iowa, which prohibits any dentist from discussing the mercury issue, we should not be surprised that its literature attempts to hide the fact that mercury is the primary component of the dental filling. The dental industry calls the fillings "silver" because it sounds benign. The filling is not benign; it is not silver but mercury. Other statements that are made in the brochure:

15

. . **"Once mercury is combined with the metals it forms a biologically inactive substance."**

Simply put it is not biologically inactive, but biologically active; Mercury vapor is released and inhaled. Dr. Svare proved this in 1980. It is absorbed by all body tissues and disrupts bodily processes at the cellular level.

. . **"Minute amounts of mercury vapor may be released . . . there is no scientific evidence that such low-level exposure is harmful."**

First replace the word *may* with *are*. It is misleading to consumers to suggest mercury may be released when the scientific community acknowledges that mercury vapor *is* released from every mercury amalgam filling. According to many studies, any exposure to any level of mercury is harmful. The ADA position, which suggests benign amounts of mercury is released, is contradicted by scientific findings. Scientists have conducted independent studies and determined that the human uptake of mercury from mercury amalgams is significant and can cause disease and death.

. . **". A few countries have suggested limiting the use of amalgam restorations in some patient populations"**

I wonder why? It is because the low level exposure causes health problems. It seems to contradict the ADA's previous statement.

. . **"There is no scientific evidence supporting a link between silver fillings and disease or chronic illnesses."**

On the contrary, there is a great deal of research that provides a connection between "silver" (mercury) fillings and Alzheimers, cancer, heart disease, M.S. and other autoimmune diseases. If this statement was written in 1890 it would have been considered unfounded. Today it is simply false.

. . **"Theoretically, a person could have an allergy to mercury, just as he could have an allergy to anything else in the environment like pollen or dust."**

This comment was written or at least approved by doctors at the ADA. Simple question: how can someone be *allergic* to a poison? Using this rationale, people could be allergic to lead, arsenic, or plutonium. Everyone reacts to mercury given a large enough exposure. Everyone dies if the exposure is large enough. If someone is exposed to a large amount of pollen or dust, they might become congested, maybe very congested, but probably will not die.

To test my theory, I called a number of allergy clinics, and told them I was allergic to mercury and could I take an antihistamine or receive allergy shots? The question was as absurd as the ADA position, but I was told that mercury was a toxic element not an allergen. I was also advised if I was exposed to mercury I should immediately call poison control or go to the closest hospital. The ADA position simply provides them an excuse should someone get sick and connect it to the mercury fillings. It is amazing that the ADA would print this brochure and hope people believe it. In this author's opinion, it is the highest form of malpractice.

If you want a copy of this brochure call the ADA at 1-800-947-4746. The brochure is called "Answers to your Questions about Silver fillings...a safe, affordable option in tooth restoration."

In a June 2001 news release, ADA president Dr. Robert Anderton asserted, "There is no sound scientific evidence supporting a link between amalgam fillings and systemic disease or chronic illness." Dr. Anderton must not read his dental journals. There are numerous published articles starting in 1957 that connect mercury escaping from amalgams into oral tissue and thus causing gum disease. Gum disease is a very serious problem. It has been repeatedly connected to heart disease. The statement by Dr. Anderton in 2001 is not true. Even ADA approved dental journals have published numerous articles on gum disease. A recent *Wall Street Journal* article, "Bacteria Behind Gum Disease are Linked to Heart Attack," describes research that strongly correlates bacteria with gum disease which then correlates to heart disease. Why would the ADA president make such a statement? As the spokesman for the dental association is he misinformed? Is gum disease not considered a chronic illness? Is the relationship between gum disease and heart disease not considered a problem? Or is he simply misleading the public? At a minimum Dr. Anderton should admit mercury amalgams are connected to heart disease. As you will discover in future sections, numerous other diseases are also connected to mercury amalgam fillings and the mercury vapor that we inhale every minute of every day that we live. The purpose of this paragraph is to simply address the daily cover-up the ADA uses to dismiss the dangers of mercury amalgams.

In summary, the vast majority of dentists use mercury amalgams to fill cavities. The ADA endorses the safety of a product that was introduced to the United States by two con men 170 years ago. The only research that has ever been done on mercury amalgams has proved that it is very dangerous and can make people very ill and, without question, damages some people's quality of life and life expectancy.

Interestingly, in the past the ADA has held mercury amalgam patents (patent #4018600 from March 14, 1978 and #4078921 from April 19, 1977). It would seem to me that this creates an obvious conflict of interest. Can the entity that controls the practices of dentists, and the entity that consumers depend on for safe and healthy dental procedures, have a financial interest in materials that are used in your mouth? How would you feel if the FDA received royalties from drug companies? It's exactly the same thing.

No company, regulatory agency, researcher or individual has ever produced research showing amalgams are *safe*. In fact, it's fair to say that if this was a new product and was presented to the FDA today for usage it would be laughed out of the system. It would never make it to phase 1 testing. Because mercury amalgams have been used for 170 years and the ADA supports its usage, nothing is being done to protect the public. The absurdity is that the FDA grandfathered the various amalgam mixtures in 1976. No testing, no scientific evidence to support their safety, and the only requirement was the fact that they had been used for a century plus and therefore received the FDA's approval for exempt status. It is a travesty and eventually will result in class action lawsuits that will make the tobacco companies seem like choirboys. It is unethical and horrific to continue to endorse and support mercury as part of any dental restoration.

Subsequent to the purported grandfathering in 1976, the U.S. Public Health Service recommended the FDA classify amalgam, and in 2002 the FDA addressed the issue. The FDA is attempting to classify mercury amalgams as Class II. Class II does not require any conditions of safety or harm to the public. The manufacturer is not required to prove safety. Consumers for Dental Choice is challenging the classification, and attempting to get mercury amalgams as a Class III product. Class III materials require the manufacturer prove the product is safe. The burden of proof must be based on peer reviewed scientific research. The FDA should mandate a Class III classification. It would finally address the mercury amalgam controversy. But the FDA knows it is impossible to prove mercury amalgams are safe; thus this is the reason for the attempt at a Class II classification.

MY STORY

I suggest readers purchase some of the books that highlight stories of patients who became ill and recovered once their mercury amalgams were removed. The best testimonial I've read is *Beating Alzheimer's* by Tom Warren. The problem I have repeating them are that I cannot attest to their validity. My information is only third-hand since the author's information is second hand. That is not to suggest these stories are not true, just that I'm uncomfortable relating them to you. However, I can provide a non-fiction story that I know is true since it's about me. From this journey through medical hell you will understand why I wrote this book.

First of all, I was 55 when this book was written. The first 40 years of my life were uneventful. Like most people of my generation I ate a well balanced diet, exercised regularly, had a successful career and two great children. I did have a history of allergies and received injections, which seemingly controlled the problems I had with pollens. In addition, I had regular physicals as part of my employment. Finally, like the majority of people in our country I believed everything a physician told me. Why not? We all have been conditioned to treat medical doctors' advice as gospel. The one thing we were not told is that all doctors are told in medical school that 50% of what they learn is not true or is subject to modification or clarification. The problem is that no one, including doctors, knows which 50% of their education is correct and which 50% is not totally accurate.

A good example of this is for decades doctors thought ulcers were caused by stress. And most people who had ulcers were doomed to a life misery since it was difficult to find a cure. Recently scientists discovered that ulcers are caused by a bacterium called helicobacter. Today medications can typically resolve ulcers in a couple of weeks. Other examples include the dangers of silicone implants, the hazards of asbestos, and the consequences of lead in paint. We continue to learn a great deal that enhances our quality of life. And our education is not over. We now know something else that is incorrect and that is the effect that mercury amalgams have on the human body. Mercury in dentistry will make some people sick. And as you will read later, mercury from your dental fillings can kill you.

Medical practitioners are not infallible. Did you know that doctors are the third leading cause of death in the United States, behind only cancer and heart disease? Unnecessary surgeries, medication mistakes, and infections in the hospital cause 250,000 deaths per year. This fact should eliminate the shield of invincibility in the medical profession. Doctors are human; they make mistakes in judgment and performance. Most doctors do not have the time to evaluate studies. They are forced to accept AMA and ADA interpretations. This is a serious problem.

Onto my saga. Fifteen years ago, I began urinating much more frequently than in the past (a very common symptom of mercury poisoning). After a few months of doing this I went to my internist and he checked me out and told me to reduce the amount of fluids I was drinking and that would reduce the frequency of urination. Interesting advice! It was rather easy to follow these instructions. I simply reduced all my intake of liquids. Subsequently I began to notice some allergies to foods. The subsequent visit to my doctor resulted with advice to simply avoid the foods I was reacting to. At this point I guess I should have asked the question regarding how tough is it to be a doctor, but I once again heeded this new advice. The next problem that arose was significant gastric problems: a lot of gas, frequent soft stools, and bouts of diarrhea. At this point a gastro specialist did numerous tests and found nothing significantly wrong. I spent 12 months discovering this enlightening diagnosis. During this time period I was prescribed antacids, which in retrospect caused as much damage as the mercury itself. This will be explained later in the book.

With no improvement I went to a new gastro "expert" with the same results. However, by this time I had many more symptoms, including severe anxiety, insomnia, canker sores, heart palpitations, tremors, itching, sore joints, fibromyalgia, memory problems, hemorrhoids, heliobactor, mycoplasma, parasites, viruses, an enlarged liver, blood sugar problems, chemical sensitivities, kidney problems, and other symptoms I'm sure I have forgotten. The only food that I could eat was white rice.

During a visit to gastro doc "#2" he decided my problems were not physical but mental so he prescribed amitriptiline, a commonly used drug to treat depression, although it also has the added effect of slowing the gastric system. After two years of seeing doctors as well as numerous specialists no one could identify a cause for the various symptoms. The various allopathic doctors suggested I see a mental health professional, maybe a shrink was the answer to my physical problems. They surmised all my problems were in my head! They had finally arrived at the correct diagnosis; the problems *were* in my head, but not the type they were prepared to treat.

In reality, the process of ongoing diarrhea was actually nature's method of trying to rid my body of toxins. Hippocrates once stated: "The natural healing force within each one of us is the greatest force in getting well." This is a statement that unfortunately, many patients and doctors have never heeded. However, the prescription drug amitriptiline ended that process since it created constipation, and now the toxins could no longer exit my body. Thus they found new homes in tissues, joints, muscles and organs which increased the severity of many symptoms, especially muscular skeletal problems. The real value of amitriptiline is to treat depression. Interestingly that is one of the only symptoms I did not have at this time. But I guess when all else fails, treat a non-existent symptom with a drug. Without doubt this was the worst possible treatment, and I believe this significantly increased the length of time it took for me to regain my health once I started treating the real problem.

The only change the prescription drug provided was diarrhea decreased but it was replaced by muscle stiffness. Every time I decided (not my doctor) to stop taking the prescription my muscle stiffness decreased and diarrhea returned. My doctor did not believe me when I made this observation and decided the solution was to increase my dosage of amitriptiline. At this point I decided I really didn't need him or the pills so I decided the only way I was going to find a solution was to do so myself. The problem with this path is that the first non-traditional approach you read that seemingly describes your symptoms is the path that you not only walk down, but also run down.

I read about being allergic to certain compounds in foods that triggered the type of symptoms that I was having and thus I found a naturopathic doctor who began desensitizing me to these compounds. One year later and thousands of dollars later I had been desensitized to 120 compounds found in food with very little change in my health. Other than this doctor taking advantage of a sick, but "I'll try anything patient," this was a total waste of time, money and energy.

The next path that I ventured down was candida. This is a very controversial subject, but there are certainly many success stores articulated in many books that give this subject creditability. I tried various candida therapies and symptoms improved a little bit. (More on this subject later.) However, please be assured that yeast overgrowth is a very real problem, and can be linked to mercury or can simply be a result of your internal ecosystem being out of balance. Birth control pills, antibiotics, and a diet that is overloaded with sugar, alcohol and yeast containing products frequently cause this unbalance. Some writers and practitioners believe candida is reaching epidemic proportions, and if addressed by mainstream medicine would result in many people with chronic illnesses being cured.

For the umpteenth time, I changed doctors and found a doctor who specialized in environmental medicine. He did a hair analysis and it showed a minor elevation in mercury. We decided to do another test to determine how much mercury my body really had in it. This second test for mercury showed somewhere between 500 and 2000 times the normal amount of mercury a person should have in their urine! The reason for the range is that different people labs and doctors have different baselines. My doctor told me this was the highest number he'd ever heard of, and I should be dead. At this level he decided I was a medical risk and he refused to treat me in any fashion.

The only source of mercury in my body was my dental fillings. All mercury amalgam fillings have at least 50% mercury as part of their metal mixture. Like all impatient and scared patients I ran to get my mercury amalgams removed. Remember, at my levels of mercury I should have been dead and since I wasn't I was probably pretty close. I got an appointment, had the mercury amalgams removed and discovered after this miserable process that I should have gotten a compatibility test done to determine what dental products I was compatible with before proceeding. Sure enough, the replacement composites I put in my mouth were comprised of cadmium, aluminum and tin. Bad move, bad product so I had to redo the entire process again.

At this point I decided that my environmental medicine doctor knew enough about mercury toxicity to diagnose it, but not enough to effectively treat it. I needed to do two things. First was to find medical professionals who were apprised of the latest research on mercury and who had effectively treated other patients. Second, I had to learn everything known to mankind on mercury toxicity so that I could be an effective patient. An effective patient does not just sit in a room and get treated like most doctors would like but asks questions, questions procedures and forces the practitioners to think. They are also willing to take certain risks and to try therapies that might prove beneficial. These are certainly not life threatening protocols but if you have a theory, try it. Remember, detoxing from mercury is still an adventure, there is no textbook solution that will work for everyone. To that end the reason for authoring this book. I want to share what I know, what pitfalls to avoid and how to detoxify generally.

The philosopher Voltaire once wrote, "Physicians pour drugs of which they know little...to cure diseases which they know less into humans which they know nothing." This described my journey toward wellness until I decided to take control of my own health.

I will state a few of my theories repeatedly in this book. These are critical as you recover from the poison that your family dentist put in your body.

.. DON'T BELIEVE TRADITIONAL MD'S REGARDING
MERCURY. They are wrong.
.. DETOXING FROM MERCURY IS A PROCESS NOT AN
EVENT. It takes time, in some cases years.
.. LEARN EVERYTHING YOU CAN FROM THIS BOOK AND
OTHER SOURCES OF INFORMATION. Become an expert.
.. DON'T GIVE UP. Stay with the process of detoxing. You will see
improvement eventually.

CHAPTER 3

Wisdom Is Supreme; Therefore Seek Wisdom

MERCURY MAKES PEOPLE SICK, MERCURY KILLS PEOPLE ... PERIOD END

The United States Department of Health and Human Services published a book entitled *Toxicological Profile for Mercury*. Buy it, borrow it, but find a way to read it. The Department of Health and Human Services states clearly that mercury is dangerous, yet the AMA and the ADA still believe that mercury is safe when placed in a person's mouth. The AMA and ADA not only continue to allow medical practitioners to poison us, but they also are constantly on witch-hunts for doctors and dentists who have holistic medical practices. If you can figure out why a book published by the United States government puts us on alert to the hazards of mercury, including mercury amalgams, and at the same time the AMA and ADA believe putting mercury in our mouths is just fine, then at a minimum you clearly understand conflicting opinions. The contradiction between the two positions is obvious; the lack of a unified position is perplexing.

As you probably learned in your high school chemistry class, mercury is a toxic liquid metal, which is volatile at room temperature. The fumes are easily inhaled, and thus absorbed into our body. Just recently I read an article about a chemistry teacher in New Hampshire who spilled a drop of mercury on her hand during a laboratory experiment and died. It was amazing that the symptoms she had during her illness are the same symptoms that many people experience from the mercury in their mercury amalgams. Needless to say, mercury is a very dangerous substance that needs to be handled with care.

The most well known source of mercury to many people is from fish. All fish contain mercury; the larger the fish, the more mercury. In fact, many mainstream traditional doctors recommend that consumers not eat fish more than a couple of times per week, and this might be too much. The reason for this is simple. By eating fish you are also consuming mercury and if you consume more mercury than you can eliminate, the result will be toxic effects.

24

A recent article stated that 40% of our nation's waters are too toxic for safe fishing. Also, these waters are too toxic to eat the fish that are caught in them. Think about this simple statement. Do you realize how much water 40% represents? This is a vast amount of toxic and polluted water. In fact, the EPA issued advisories for more than 1500 rivers, bays and lakes in 1995. The reason for most of these advisories is mercury contamination. The EPA provides information on many symptoms that will occur in people who eat mercury toxic fish. Guess what? These are the same symptoms that present themselves in people who are poisoned by mercury amalgams.

In 1997, David Brown prepared a mercury study for the Northeast and parts of Canada. He concluded that a pregnant woman who ate only one fish from the tested waterways would consume enough mercury to harm a fetus.

The most famous case of mercury poisoning from fish occurred in Minamata, Japan. Thousands of individuals became sick from eating fish with elevated levels of methyl mercury, (remember from a previous section methyl mercury is the most toxic form of mercury) and over 100 people died. This bit of history seems to have been disregarded science, and even more frightening is that from this tragedy we also learned that mercury can penetrate the placental membrane in pregnant women, thus affecting the fetus. The name "Fetal Minamata Disease" was used to identify children affected by mercury and who were born with a number of maladies including cerebral palsy. Tragically, many children born with Fetal Minamata Disease died. From this we might hypothesize that some cases of cerebral palsy may be connected to mercury passing from the mom to the fetus. It would seem that research dollars should be spent researching this possible connection.

In November 1997 the United States government stated that pregnant women who consume large amounts of fish could pass mercury and its toxicity to their fetus. The study was done on more than 900 seven year olds born to women from the Faroe Islands. The fish consumed by these women came from the North Atlantic Ocean near Scotland. The study concluded a relationship between neurological damage in children and exposure to mercury during pregnancy. The study generally concluded that mercury "builds up" in fish and can affect children of pregnant women who eat the fish. Just recently *20/20* did a segment on its popular television show stating that pregnant women should not eat fish with elevated mercury. The risk to the fetus is too great.

In 2001 R. Goldman wrote in the *American Academy of Pediatrics*, "The developing fetus and young children are thought to be disproportionately affected by mercury exposure because many aspects of development, particularly brain maturation, can be disturbed by the presence of mercury. Minimizing mercury exposure is therefore essential to optimal child health."

In 1969 the FDA published acceptable levels for mercury in fish of 0.5 parts per million. In 1979 the guideline doubled to 1.0 ppm after the fishing industry sued. In 1998 Congress asked the National Academy of Sciences (NAS) to research mercury levels in fish. Mercury levels in swordfish, shark and tuna were consistently above the FDA guidelines of 1 ppm. The range of mercury accumulation for these fish was significant; at the high end swordfish was 3.73 ppm, shark was 4.45 ppm, and tuna 1.3 ppm. The group with the greatest risk from high levels of mercury is pregnant women according to NAS. Even a level of 1 ppm may expose a fetus to neurological problems such as lower IQ's and learning disabilities.

An article in the *Oakland Tribune* on December 2, 2002 detailed the problems Bay Area waterways have with mercury. During the gold rush era the problem with mercury in rivers, streams, and bays developed. An estimated 26 million pounds of mercury were used to extract gold from dirt and gravel. The process of using mercury to extract gold was stopped in 1884. But the damage was already done. A huge quantity of mercury escaped into the environment, and mercury just does not go away. All 26 million pounds of mercury has found a home in local waterways. Seasonal rains caused the mercury to flow into rivers and eventually the San Francisco Bay. As we already know, methyl mercury in aquatic environments poses serious problems; it is easily absorbed and difficult to eliminate. Jim Weiner, an expert on mercury in fish, stated, "the concentrations (of mercury) in fish are often times a million to ten million times what you see in water."

The EPA guideline for mercury is 0.1 microgram per kilogram of body weight per day. According to the EPA, below this level there are no adverse health effects from ingested mercury. This is not a lot of mercury. According to the EPA, if this threshold is abused, then adverse health effects can be the result. The EPA estimates that 7% of women

26

nationwide exceed this limit. Using this as a guideline, approximately 60,000 babies born each year are at risk for mercury toxicity.

The EPA stated that women exposed to mercury vapor experience greater hormonal disturbances and more spontaneous abortions than women not exposed. In addition there is a higher mortality rate among infants born to women who displayed symptoms of mercury toxicity.

Mercury poses serious consequences for a fetus. Three facts are known: 1) mercury passes through the placenta and becomes part of the fetus's development; 2) mercury that a pregnant woman absorbs can come from air, fish or amalgams; 3) mercury can affect DNA.

Once fertilization takes place mercury can interfere with a person's DNA. Each partner contributes 23 pair of chromosomes. Mercury can alter the entire process and produce 22 or 24 or alter any pair of chromosomes. Researchers found a relationship between mercury in the blood and chromosome alterations. And mercury in the blood corresponds to the number of mercury amalgams in a person's mouth. Research has also demonstrated that a fetus can accumulate 8 to 30 times more mercury than its mother. A fetus has almost no mechanism to eliminate mercury, which leads to accumulation. It is possible for a fetus to be poisoned at conception. This results in DNA alterations or during pregnancy, from mercury passing through the placenta.

Any pediatrician will agree that neither parent should be mercury toxic at the time of conception. – the risk to the fetus is too great; however, pediatricians just do not believe that mercury can come from dental amalgams. In spite of this traditional view, the American Pediatric Association advises physicians to recommend mercury free dentists to parents concerned about their child's exposure to mercury.

An interesting fact: birth defects are up 500% since 1940. Why? Health and knowledge of health is better today than 60 years ago, pediatricians are more knowledgeable than 60 years ago, and hospitals are more qualified than 60 years ago. Why the increase in birth defects? I bet that pregnant moms have more mercury amalgams and eat more fish than 60 years ago. Fish has been labeled a healthy alternative to meat, and far more fish is consumed today versus a few decades ago. Thus more mercury is absorbed and passed to the fetus.

In addition to the problems mercury causes during pregnancy, mercury has also been associated with low sperm counts and the inability for a contaminated egg to be fertilized. This is probably nature's method of avoiding birth defects. Nevertheless, infertility is on the rise in the 21st century. This is another trend that seems backward given today's environment versus 60 years ago.

In addition to the problem of mercury in fish we have also seen the use of mercury in industrial and agricultural applications increase. There are numerous examples of people becoming ill and even dying from eating food treated with mercury as part of a fungicide.

Currently the EPA is researching standards for coal fired utility boilers. The rules should be in place by 2004 and trigger a reduction in air born mercury. This industry releases 40 tons of mercury annually in the United States. It is released into the air we breathe and water we drink.

In discussing new regulations for power plants, EPA administrator Carol Bowen stated in a 1998 EPA study that mercury was the most serious health hazard of all the pollutants. Mercury is not broken down by nature or any metabolic process but transforms into methyl mercury and collects in the fatty tissues of fish. Ultimately that mercury ends up in those who eat fish. Assuming Bowen is correct, can we assume that mercury vapor that is inhaled by everyone who has mercury amalgams also transforms into methyl mercury and is deposited in our fatty tissue? The answer is yes.

The events of the tragedy of September 11th significantly elevated mercury levels at Ground Zero. Four New York policemen working at the site discovered they had elevated blood mercury levels. The fact that their blood levels were elevated indicates that the exposure was recent. According to health officials, a blood level of 13 micrograms per liter of blood is acceptable and the 4 officers had measured levels of 14, 14, 18 and 24. In all probability the mercury source was mercury from fluorescent light bulbs. Depending on the size of the light bulb, each fluorescent bulb contains approximately 25-65 milligrams of mercury. Assuming thousands of lights were destroyed, that represents a great deal of mercury that was released into the air. This contamination as well as any new mercury dental fillings would cause a serious elevation in blood mercury levels.

Although fluorescent light bulbs are energy efficient they contain mercury. Thus, if they break in your house they need to be dealt with very carefully. When they finally no longer emit light they need to be disposed of as toxic waste. Many states have laws regarding special procedures for fluorescent lights. Those states that do not have laws should. Simply put, they should not be placed in normal trash that is placed in landfills. As a consumer you should not purchase fluorescent lights regardless of the energy savings because the risk that one will break in your home far offsets the energy savings.

So now we come to mercury and your local dentist. The history of the mercury amalgam was discussed in the previous chapter. Many authors describe the history of mercury using *amalgam wars*. The wars are being waged between the scientific community and the dental community. In the early and mid 1800's the use of mercury in amalgams was banned by a predecessor organization to the ADA. The reason: mercury was a poison, and the original dental society did not want a material used that caused illness, disease and death. It is rather appropriate and compassionate to have an organization care about its constituent's health. Also, it is rather novel considering the events of today. Unfortunately this was just the beginning of the mercury debates that continue to the present day. The group eventually spilt over the mercury issue. During the next century the use of mercury amalgams grew due to their simplicity and cost, and they became the dental material of choice used in dentists' offices.

In 1926 the mercury controversy once again surfaced *(the second amalgam war)* based on the scientific findings of Dr. Stock. Dr. Stock stated that mercury was dangerous in dental fillings. The mercury vapor created made people sick. As expected, this created the next controversy, the next set of opinions and fortunately more research. Then in the early 1980's, additional research on mercury amalgams and mercury in dental fillings led to some major breakthroughs that have continued until today *(the third amalgam war)*.

Currently many countries have limited or dramatically reduced the use of mercury fillings; these include Switzerland, Sweden, Austria, Norway, Japan, Germany, France and Canada. Amalgams are contraindicated in the following countries in certain situations: Sweden, Germany, Austria, Canada, and the United Kingdom. Sweden, German, Austria, and Canada recommend an amalgam-free mouth for children. Germany recommends no mercury amalgams if kidney disease exists. It is clear that many countries do not want mercury amalgams in their citizen's mouths. Why would any one want to use them, particularly when great nontoxic options are available that will not create health risks?

Numerous states within the United States are addressing the mercury issue; these include California, Arizona, Alabama, Georgia, Illinois, Iowa, Maine, New Hampshire, Ohio, and Oregon. In addition the National Black Caucus of State Legislators have called for an end to mercury in dental restorations. Finally, HR 4165 introduced by Congresswoman Diane Watson and Congressman Dan Burton would eventually eliminate mercury in all dental material.

Many dentists in the United States have mercury-free practices, much to the chagrin of the ADA. Finally, we have medical doctors and clinics that exist to treat mercury toxic patients. Why has this taken so long? And why in the United States are we still fighting and arguing over this issue?

First of all I know mercury in dental fillings can make people sick. It made me sick. Second, the AMA and the ADA also know this fact – too many people have made them aware, and there is too much research to prove this point. Why does the AMA and ADA deny the dangers of mercury? Could it be that if they admitted this that the "fallout" from it would be costly? How many health conscious consumers would want their fillings removed and replaced with healthy alternatives? Or better put who wouldn't want them removed? Who would pay for this procedure, insurance companies? How many sick people who are sick without any hope would pursue this avenue? Finally, and maybe most importantly, how many lawsuits would result from people who were poisoned by their dentists with total approval and support from the AMA and the ADA? Remember we have become a very litigious society. This could get awfully expensive for many individuals and groups, including dentists, doctors, insurance companies, malpractice entities, the AMA and the ADA and anyone else someone could include in their litigation.

Thus far it appears no entity is warning the public regarding the dangers of mercury amalgams. The ADA strongly defends the product, the local dentist believes the ADA and every regulatory entity also supports the usage of mercury as a dental restoration. But manufacturers of mercury amalgams provide warnings about their product. The MSDS (Material Safety Data Sheet) for Dispersalloy, a manufacturer of a popular mercury amalgam, states its product should not be used in children under six or by pregnant women. The MSDS also indicates that mercury amalgams should not be used on anyone with kidney disease. Another MSDS warning states that mercury has been reported to be associated with a variety of health effects, including reproductive toxicity. These warnings are ignored by most dentists. In my opinion, a lawsuit should be filed by every parent of a child under six who has a mercury amalgam in his or her mouth. Ditto for every pregnant woman. This qualifies as malpractice. The manufacturer issued a warning and is being ignored by the dentist, the user of the product.

Succinctly, *when* not *if*, the fact that mercury amalgams make people sick is acknowledged (it has already been proven), a number of entities are at real financial risk. I no longer own any stock in health insurance organizations. Financially they cannot absorb the expense associated with the plethora of risks forthcoming. Finally, in this country we are superb at trauma care. If someone is in an accident, or has a heart attack, we do a great job at sustaining life. However our system fails us miserably when it comes to prevention. Doctors treat numerous symptoms but seldom ever try to find the cause: mercury. Once we address this fact maybe we can make inroads into the war on mercury amalgams.

Numerous symptoms result from the absorbed mercury from dental fillings. Most of these symptoms are treated with a drug by traditional doctors. Until the underlying cause is addressed we are simply masking symptoms with prescription drugs that cause additional problems, i.e., side effects on top of mercury poisoning.

At the beginning of this chapter, I related the fact that a pregnant mom with mercury amalgams will release mercury, which will be absorbed by her fetus. Why would anyone do this willingly? Why would anyone who is hoping to give birth someday work in environments where mercury is present, eat food contaminated by mercury, or have mercury fillings? The source of the mercury is irrelevant. Mercury from any source causes fetal damage. Basically everyone that is doing this is rolling the dice – will it affect my child or not? Will it affect him or her at birth or years later? It is a stupid bet. Mercury harms the child just like it harms you. Have you wondered why, in the last century, so many childhood "malfunctions" exist? Why has the incidence of childhood leukemia increased so much during the past few decades? Or how about attention deficits disorder - this was never heard of 25 years ago. More and more kids are on Ritalin? Why? Or how about SIDS? There are already articles that demonstrate a relationship between SIDS and mercury. One of the most compelling facts is that when Australia stopped many mandatory vaccines, its SIDS rate dropped dramatically.

I hope that medical research asks these same questions and considers the impact mercury has in all areas of the human body. We deserve the opportunity to be healthy, and most parents work very hard to insure good health for their child. I believe that the AMA and ADA are sabotaging our efforts. I hope that everyone that reads this book, if they do not get their own mercury amalgams removed, certainly demand that their children receive composite fillings and not mercury amalgams.

If the assessment that we are currently in an amalgam war is correct, then it is time that this *war* is brought to a conclusion once and for all. Since the early 1800s it has been known that mercury amalgams are dangerous and should not be used. In the last 175 years additional research continues to support this hypothesis. There is no research to support the safety of mercury amalgams. It is time to end this debate and correct the cover-ups, the misinformation and the lies promulgated by the ADA and the AMA.

The bottom line is that mercury fillings cause people to get sick and die. This affects many people. Maybe you are one of them. And one final thought: why do dentists die so young? Why do dentist commit suicide at the highest rate of any profession? Why do dentists have the highest divorce rate of any profession? Is it because they have such a stressful job or that they are breathing mercury fumes all day year after year? Research has demonstrated that the average age at the time of death for a dentist is late 50's or early 60's. Think about what you just read – this is compelling. I think the first place you should distribute this book is to your dentist. Assuming your dentist has an open mind and has not been brainwashed by the ADA, this will either save his/her life or at a minimum extend their life.

Dr. Henry Schroeder, professor Emeritus at Dartmouth University Medical School wrote in his book *The Poisons Around Us*, "Cadmium, mercury, lead, beryllium, and antimony are involved in at least half the deaths in the United States and much of the disabling disease."

Remember the four practical issues for obtaining good health:

. . DON'T BELIEVE TRADITIONAL MD'S REGARDING MERCURY. They are wrong.
. . DETOXING FROM MERCURY IS A PROCESS, NOT AN EVENT. It takes time, in some cases years.
. . LEARN EVERYTHING YOU CAN FROM THIS BOOK AND OTHER SOURCES OF INFORMATION. Become an expert.
. . DON'T GIVE UP. Stay with the process of detoxifying. You will see improvement eventually.

CHAPTER 4

When Pride Comes, Then Comes Disgrace, But With Humility Comes Wisdom

STUDIES PROVING AMALAGAMS ARE DANGEROUS

DR. STOCK'S RESEARCH

One of the first people to recognize the dangers of mercury amalgams was Dr. Alfred Stock of Germany in 1936. He was ill and determined his problems were the result of mercury vapors being released from his dental fillings. He ultimately diagnosed his own problem; he was mercury toxic. Dr. Stock published the process of mercury poisoning, calling it a creeping illness. He condemned the use of mercury amalgams. In different times his research might have changed history, saved lives and improved the quality of life for millions, but his research and laboratory were destroyed in Second World War. Fortunately, Dr. Stock planted a seed. Others investigated his research and arrived at the same conclusion; mercury is very toxic to anyone who is exposed to it.

DR. VIMY'S RESEARCH

The most important study and work took place in Calgary, Alberta, Canada, in the early 1980's. It proved mercury is released from dental amalgams and through inhalation is deposited in various organs. Dr. Vimy used radioactive mercury as a dental filling on six sheep. The reason radioactive mercury was used was to insure that any mercury findings were not confused with daily environmental mercury intake and to X-ray the path the mercury might take if it was released from the dental cavity. The sheep's mercury amalgams were on the top back molars where most of the chewing occurs. After only three days, the sheep had mercury in their droppings. After 29 days, X-rays were taken and the radioactive mercury was in every organ.

The greatest concentrations were in the brain, kidney, liver and GI track. The most interesting aspect of the study was that the concentrations of mercury in both the urine and the blood of the sheep were not significant.

Concentrations in the kidney were 700 times more than in the blood. In other words, mercury was storing in the kidney and not releasing in urine. The primary exit of mercury was through the feces. Other organs with seriously elevated levels were the stomach, the liver and gum tissue. This study proved a number of facts regarding amalgams:

1. **Mercury is released from amalgams.**
2. **Mercury vapor is inhaled and deposited in every organ in the body.**
3. **Kidneys retain mercury and thus the need for a mechanism (a chelating agent) to eliminate it.**
4. **The feces is the primary avenue for the elimination of mercury.**

This research should have been the starting point for change. The discovery was dramatic and conclusive. Amazingly, this research was criticized by the dental society because sheep chew differently than humans. This is true but the facts were still undeniable. Instead of the dental profession pursuing this information and determining the validity, they dismissed the research because of chewing techniques. Their objective was not science and research but the desire to defend the practice of using mercury amalgams.

Dr. Vimy decided to duplicate the process with a monkey. Results were similar, after 28 days mercury was present in every organ. Deposits of mercury were different in various organs and most importantly larger amounts of mercury were present in the GI track and the liver. Depending on the interpretation, the monkey absorbed more mercury than the sheep. The monkey chewed in a similar manner when compared to humans. So it was easy to dismiss the absurd chew excuse. The dental profession now had research that should have caused an immediate ban on mercury amalgams.

Dr. Vimy did another study to evaluate kidney function. He had both a control group, i.e. no mercury amalgams and a test group, i.e. with mercury amalgams. Sheep were used in this evaluation. Suffice to say the control group had no change in kidney function. The sheep with mercury amalgams showed a 54% reduction in kidney function after 30 days and a 60% reduction after 60 days. Two additional findings showed that sodium in urine from the control group tripled and protein excretion (albumin) dropped 33% from the norm.

The interesting correlation to the above finding is that most mercury toxic patients have below normal sodium levels. This will demonstrate itself in two different tests: hair analysis, and fecal analysis. Sodium level is an excellent indicator of mercury toxicity.

In spite of Vimy's research over 20 years ago, mercury amalgams are still being used by 98% of dentists. This seems to be not only ignorant but also malpractice.

CONTROL STUDY OF 1569 PATIENTS AND SYMPTOMS

A study by the Foundation for Toxic Free Dentistry of 1569 patients who had their mercury amalgams removed illustrates the dramatic changes that can occur when mercury is removed from your mouth. The individuals had a variety of symptoms and were asked to respond positively or negatively if that symptom changed after mercury amalgam removal. The following is a partial list.

Symptom	% improvement after amalgam removal
Lack of energy	97
Gum problems	94
Anxiety	93
Depression	91
Allergies	89
Temper	89
Headaches and migraines	87
Thyroid problems	79
MS symptoms	76

This study indicated many other symptoms also improved. The above list, however, is indicative of the problems many people struggle with every day. These are maladies that medical doctors treat daily. Most shrinks earn a six-figure income by prescribing drugs for some of these "medical conditions." As a consumer do you think the medical community has this type of success rate with prescription drugs? I have not seen a similar survey but I highly doubt it.

- For instance, what current AMA protocol increases energy by 97% in all patients that are treated?

- *Newsweek* recently suggested that 13% of our population suffers from anxiety. According to this survey removing mercury amalgams will help 93% of these individuals. This is a drug free solution to a vexing and expensive societal problem.

- Various studies state that 30-50% of our population suffers daily from depression. Does Prozac work in 91% of people taking the drug for depression?

- Do allergy shots or antihistamines improve 89% of allergy patients?

- Does Nuprin, Aleve, Tylenol or Advil relieve 87% of headaches, including migraines?

- What M.S. drugs improve 76% of M.S. patients?

- Would you prefer a synthetic thyroid hormone or have an amalgam free mouth in order to improve thyroid function?

- How can our society reduce physical abuse, road rage, and other forms of anger management in 89% of people? As you will hear later in the book, mercury is a neurotoxin and is shown to cause anger, rage and other forms of violent behavior.

Assuming this sample of 1569 represents a cross section of our population, removing mercury amalgams can create a massive change in our quality of life. How would you like to own stock in a company that could accomplish the above changes? It would be a hot stock. The good news is that as a consumer, it costs very little to receive the benefit of this perceived "stock." Simply replace your mercury dental fillings. The dividend you receive is a vastly improved quality of life.

It is interesting to understand the vicious cycle that occurs when mainstream medicine treats the above symptoms, but not the cause. Most drugs that are prescribed create a new side effect that is dry mouth or reduced saliva. These drugs are Prozac, Xanax, Valium, Lopressor, Inasotec, antihistimines, and acme medications etc. Saliva is a natural antibiotic. Less saliva, via prescription drugs, equals more bacteria in the mouth. This causes more decay; more decay equals more mercury fillings. This leads more toxicity and therefore more symptoms. The cycle is never ending until some type of disease causes death.

THE COORS STUDY

The Coors Study funded by The Coors Foundation (yes the same company that makes beer) decided to test the effect of mercury amalgams on various blood chemistries. In order to control the process, 27 individuals were chosen who had three to ten mercury amalgam fillings and no root canals, metal crowns, bridges or braces. This control insured that other heavy metals were not going to influence the study. They were tested four times: before any dental work was done, i.e. with mercury amalgams, after the mercury amalgams were removed, after mercury amalgams were reinserted in the mouth and finally after mercury amalgams were removed a second time. When mercury amalgams were removed the following findings were documented.

1. 91% of the patients had a drop in their white blood count
2. T lymphocytes normalized
3. Hemoglobin levels dropped in 22 patients but energy levels increased
4. Oxygen saturation in the blood increased from 43% to 57% (norm is 75-80%)

Findings one and two illustrate that the immune system is recovering from a battle with mercury. We can conclude that mercury seriously impacts the immune system; once mercury is removed, however, the immune system is able to effectively recover.

Findings three and four are worth evaluating. This suggests elevated hemoglobin is possibly a signal of toxicity. In theory, as hemoglobin loses oxygen, and the oxygen is replaced by mercury, the body makes more hemoglobin. The body cannot rid itself of the mercury so it produces more hemoglobin to compensate. When the mercury is no longer a threat, i.e. it is removed from the individual's mouth, the need for extra hemoglobin is no longer necessary and the body now produces less hemoglobin. Simultaneously, oxygen finds a binding site on the hemoglobin and oxygen saturation increases. Thus it is not the amount of hemoglobin that is important but the amount of oxygen that binds to the hemoglobin that is critical. This will be discussed in greater detail in a subsequent chapter.

5. After mercury amalgam removal 17 patients showed drops in levels of prophyrin from an average of 416 to 58 mcg.

Prophyrin breaks down into heme. Two processes take place at this point. One, the heme combines with globin to form hemoglobin, and two it creates ATP our primary source of energy. When prophyrin metabolism is altered the above processes are compromised and prophyrins are discarded in the urine. When mercury is present elevated levels are found in the urine. Elevated prophyrin levels (over 300 mcg) are a strong indicator of mercury toxicity. For example, an M.S. patient had prophyrin levels above 2100; after removing the mercury amalgams the level dropped to 200. One of the biggest challenges in evaluating prophyrin levels is finding a laboratory that can accurately test prophyrin levels because most are not qualified to measure these levels. If a laboratory in your area can effectively measure prophyrin levels, this is an excellent test to determine the potential for mercury toxicity. However, the method of collection and the technology must allow for an accurate measurement.

Prophyrin, like oxygen, is a source of energy. If oxygen is reduced and prophyrin is lost in the urine, the common symptom is fatigue. The symptom does not change until blood chemistries are altered. Blood chemistries do not change until the source of the mercury is eliminated.

The Coors Study in 1998 is another in the list of valuable research that proves the serious harm mercury amalgams cause.

BOYD HALEY'S RESEARCH ON MERCURY AMALGAM VAPOR

Boyd Haley has conducted extensive research on the toxicity of mercury from mercury amalgams. The ADA claims the mercury amalgam surfaces give off 0.067 to 0.057 micrograms of mercury/day/square cm of surface. No research to support this "fact." Haley concluded from his research the release is 7.54 micrograms of mercury/day/square cm of surface and 45.49 micrograms of mercury/day/square cm of surface when brushing with a medium bristle toothbrush. The discrepancy between the ADA position and Haley's research is 750 times greater release of mercury.

NATIONAL INSTITUTE OF DENTAL RESEARCH

NIDR is a government sponsored research facility responsible for determining dental product compatibility. Common sense would suggest that mercury amalgam research would be high on their list of priorities, but until recently it was never analyzed. In 1999 NIDR did a study on 1127 seemingly healthy males. The purpose of the study was to determine mercury concentrations in the blood and urine associated with mercury amalgams.

The age of the group was 40-78 years with an average age of 52.8. The range of mercury amalgam surfaces was 0-66 (66 is a lot amalgams surfaces!), with an average of 20 surfaces. As a note, this sample represents more mercury amalgam surfaces than a traditional cross section of our population. This is probably due to the age, gender, and vocation of the subjects. The average mercury secreted in the urine of men with mercury amalgams was 4.5 micrograms per day. Those with over 49 mercury amalgam surfaces averaged in excess 8.7 micrograms per day. The portion of the study with no mercury amalgam surfaces secreted virtually no mercury. This supports the fact that the mercury originated from amalgams. The study did not evaluate elimination through the intestines or sweat, but if it was measured it would be fair to state the 4.5 and the 8.7 micrograms are baseline amounts not total excretion. Over 90% of the mercury in the urine was inorganic mercury the type that originates in mercury amalgams not fish. The EPA guideline is 6.0 micrograms. The interesting question is why isn't the guideline zero? Why is it acceptable to have any levels of mercury? The goal should be elimination and not tolerance of a safe hypothetical guideline!

At this point the study has not provoked any further action. The purpose of the study was simply to measure mercury levels in urine of those with and without mercury amalgams. It is clear from the study that NIDR has proven mercury from amalgams is released, inhaled and some of it exits via the kidney. It is also a fact that depending on the number of mercury amalgams some individuals exceed the EPA guideline. In addition if NIDR used a chelator to stimulate additional release of mercury the numbers would have been much higher, and in the group with 49 plus mercury amalgam surfaces, significantly higher. Remember, Vimy's research suggests mercury is retained in the kidney with only small amounts released in the urine. Thus the amount measured in the study is only the portion that is being released not the total burden. Let us hope some responsible agency, perhaps the Surgeon General's Office, decides to pursue this valuable research.

VETERANS ADMINISTRATION STUDY

In the 1960s the Veterans Administration studied over 1000 outwardly healthy men. The portion of the study that had gum disease suffered twice the death rate of those without periodontal disease, i.e., the group with healthy gums. The primary reason for death was cardiovascular disease. The conclusion of the study was "gum disease kills – floss or die." The conclusion is correct. The symptom is gum disease. The cause of gum disease was ignored in the study. No one correlated mercury amalgams with gum disease. Future studies since have determined mercury fillings are the primary cause for periodontal disease. Using this information it is not difficult to hypothesize mercury amalgams may increase a person's risk for heart disease.

TUBINGEN STUDY

In 1995 mercury levels in the saliva of 17500 German participants were related to the number of mercury amalgams in their mouth. Approximately 43% had mercury levels that exceeded the World Health Organization's tolerable levels. This study correlated increased mercury levels in the saliva with the following symptoms: bleeding gums, metallic taste in the mouth, impaired memory, insomnia, nervousness, and gastrointestinal problems.

OTHER VALUABLE STUDIES

- Dr. W. N. Deliargyris of the University of North Carolina confirmed earlier studies that correlate gum disease and heart disease. In the study, he discovered that 85% of heart attack patients also had periodontal disease. This is another in a long line of studies that suggest periodontal disease is a precursor of potential heart problems. One cause of periodontal disease is mercury amalgams.

- In November 1998, 20 manic depressed individuals were assessed as it related to mercury amalgams. Eleven of the 20 had their mercury amalgams removed, nine had plastic put over the mercury amalgams. After eight months the symptoms of the eleven bipolar individuals who had their mercury amalgams removed showed improvement. The nine without replacements were the same. No chelators were used; no vitamins and mineral protocols were used. The changes were due to the removal of the mercury. No one has used this small sample or the outcome to do further research. But the implications are huge as it relates to mental health conditions.

- In 1992, Berlin, et al, exposed pregnant squirrel monkeys to mercury vapor. The results demonstrated aberrant pregnancies, including premature births, lower birth weights and increased abortions.

- In 1994 the University of Munich evaluated tissues of babies who died from SIDS. The baby's tissue levels correlated with the number of mercury amalgams in their mother's mouth. We know that mercury passes from mom to the fetus. Based on this one study Germany issued an advisory against mercury amalgams in all females who are of childbearing age. Why did this information never cross the Atlantic Ocean? Maybe it did, but our politicians and regulatory agencies chose to ignore it. The horrible tragedy of this decision is that lives have been lost and the pain of a child's death is never removed. It could have been avoided if we performed a similar study. We could have arrived at the same conclusion.

- Oskarsson in 1996 confirmed that mercury from amalgams was the main source of mercury in breast milk. Thus breast-feeding from a mother with mercury amalgams is another source of mercury to an infant.

- Dr. Eggelston studied the effects of mercury amalgams and he believes that mercury reduces our immune function from one-half to one-third. Thus mercury amalgams compromise our immune system and the implications for disease, and particularly, autoimmune diseases cannot be ignored. Again, the best description of mercury is a slow leak, a slow poison that eventually demonstrates itself in a variety of ways.

- The work of Professor Skave of Sweden resulted in two important conclusions. First, mercury is eliminated at a rate at least 20 times greater in fecal matter than urine. This suggests it is valuable to have a high fiber diet and use other methodologies to increase transit time in the intestines. Second, numerous mercury amalgams in a person's mouth showed mercury excretion 100 times greater than if mercury existed only from normal external daily exposure. Conclusion: mercury is leaking from amalgams and can be eliminated with the proper protocols, from some organs but probably not from others without a chelating agent. A chelating agent is a drug that binds mercury for elimination.

- Autopsy studies in Sweden showed that the pituitary glands of dentists held more than 800 times more mercury than non-dentists. From previous research we know that both the pituitary gland and the thyroid have a very high affinity for mercury. This study should not be surprising since dentists breathe mercury vapor all day in the preparation of mercury amalgams. The pituitary strongly influences emotions, such as depression, anxiety etc. With this much mercury residing in a critical brain gland is it surprising dentists are first in the following?
  - highest suicide rates
  - highest divorce rates
  - earliest average age of death
  - highest utilization of health insurance claims
  - highest spontaneous abortions occur in the dental profession

No studies have been done to evaluate the incidence of cancer, heart disease, M.S. or other autoimmune disease, but I believe it is good bet dentists are very high on those lists as well.

- A recent study indicated a slight imbalance in thyroid hormones during pregnancy damages a fetus neurologically and consistently produces reduced IQ's in a child. A source of thyroid imbalance is mercury. Mercury has a strong affinity for the thyroid gland.

- In 1993 Anne Summers, a molecular biologist at the University of Georgia, demonstrated how bacteria in both the intestines and the mouth develop resistance to antibiotics due to the presence of mercury. The primary source of the mercury, according to Summers is the dental amalgam. In April 1993 the *New York*

Times chronicled Summers research. The interesting aspect of the research is that today's antibiotics cannot destroy bacteria mutated in the presence of mercury. There was no response by the ADA, AMA or the Surgeon General. Health care users ignored the research, and the only response by drug companies was to develop better antibiotics. The medical concern regarding the overuse of antibiotics and the fact that some bacteria are resistant to current drugs is alarming. Someone should revisit this research.

- Researchers at the Maurice Lamontagne Institute and the Swedish University of Agricultural Sciences proved that mercury passes through the blood brain barrier and enters the brain. The blood brain membrane prevents some toxins, in circulating blood, from infiltrating the brain. But the membrane is not effective against mercury. The researchers exposed two groups of trout to mercury. One group of fish had mercury added to their tank; the other fish were injected with mercury. The fish in the contaminated water had mercury accumulate in their brain, the fish injected with mercury showed no brain mercury. The speculation is that mercury traveled via the mouth through the olfactory nerves to the brain. Dr. Rouleau at the National Water Research Institute suggested mercury can accumulate in the human brain via nerve transport. The implication for neurological disease is obvious.

- Vimy and Lorsheider discovered that individuals with mercury amalgams had nine times more mercury vapor in their oral cavity than individuals without mercury amalgams. When they chewed these same individuals had a six-fold increase in mercury vapor. Thus individuals with mercury amalgams had 54 times more mercury in their oral cavity when chewing than individuals without mercury amalgams.

- Researchers from the Department of Environmental Medicine at the University of Rochester in New York determined the NAC (a glutathione precursor) significantly increases urinary methyl mercury excretion, as much as 10 times normal.

- A study of 98 dentists and a control group of 54 non-dentists revealed a significant difference in neuro behavioral tests. The dentists had an average exposure to mercury amalgams of 5.5 years. The dentists performed worse on all the following tests:

finger tapping, visual scanning, motor coordination and concentration, verbal and visual memory, and coordination speed. The performance also suggested the longer exposure to mercury the poorer the performance in the neuro behavioral tests.

- In 2002, 180 dentists were studied at the Royal Glasgow Infirmary in Scotland. They were found to have four times more mercury in their urine and nails as well as more kidney and memory problems than the general public.

- A John Hopkins University study determined that high levels of mercury in toenails correlated with an increased risk of heart disease.

- Cornett et al discovered elevated levels of mercury in people with Alzheimer's.

- In an article published in the *New England Journal of Medicine*, Clarkson stated mercury causes kidney and liver impairment as well as neurological symptoms.

- A German study concluded that mercury excretion is reduced by 5 times after removal of amalgams.

- A Finnish study correlated the number of dental amalgams with an increased risk of acute myocardial function.

- In 1994 Rowland studied the fertility of females in the dental industry. In evaluating 418 female dental assistants and comparing them to an unexposed control group he concluded they were less fertile than females working in an environment devoid of mercury.

- In 1998 Sandbough and Englund continued to validate the fact that inhaled mercury is absorbed in a person's body. They exposed volunteers to 400 ug of mercury vapor for 15 minutes. 69% of the mercury was retained; there was a rapid absorption in the blood and plasma. In the first 3 days 1% was excreted in the urine, over 30 days there was a wide range of excretion, between 8% and

40%. It does not take a math major to determine a lot of mercury remained in the body after the testing period.

- A study published in the *Journal of Dental Research* conducted by Sandbough and Englund concluded, "The process of removing amalgam fillings can have a considerable impact of mercury levels in biological fluids."

- Nylander autopsied three dentists and discovered the mercury level in their renal cortex ranged from .945 to 2.110. In a control group the range was .021-.810. No mention was made of mercury amalgams in either group. At the low end of the range the difference was 4400% more mercury in the dentist and at the high end 150% more mercury.

- A study of zinc determined a high incidence of zinc deficiency in people with ADD, autism, depression, schizophrenic, and bipolar disorders. Zinc deficiency and mercury toxicity go hand in hand.

- A study by Blumer in Australia analyzed 80 people with dental amalgams who exhibited symptoms associated with mercury toxicity. Using a chelator to stimulate mercury removal, the study concluded those with mercury amalgams had significantly higher mercury levels in their urine than those without mercury amalgams. The 80 individuals had their amalgams removed and continued to use chelators to remove mercury. In 90 days the patients were either improved, or in some cases, symptom free.

- A National Institute of Health study suggests that 90% of the elemental mercury in the body is from mercury amalgams, not fish.

Additional studies are mentioned later in the book when individual diseases associated with mercury are discussed.

The general conclusion that can be drawn from all these studies is that mercury enters the blood stream via the lungs and oral membranes; it is then distributed to every cell, tissue, and organ in the human body; and the blood brain barrier is no barrier for mercury and mercury enters the brain.

In order to combat the plethora of studies that conclude that there are dangers from mercury amalgams, the ADA published the following statement in the *Journal of American Dental Association* (April 1990): "The strongest and most convincing support we have for the safety of the dental amalgam is the fact that each year more than 100 million amalgam fillings are placed in the United States. Since amalgam has been used for more than 150 years, literally billions of amalgam fillings have been successfully used to restore decayed teeth." No science to support its usage, just history. As a consumer are your decisions based on historical reference, or research and science? The tragedy of the above statement is that no one challenged the ADA to refute the plethora of studies that contradict its policy statement. No one wanted proof.

CHANGING PARADIGM

The generation prior to ours believed everything the family doctor said. The family doctor was revered. However, the generation reading this book has altered the prior trend. Here are a few facts that reveal a generation that challenges traditional allopathic concepts:

1)   In 1997 Americans made 627 million visits to alternative practitioners, visits to traditional doctors numbered 386 million.
2)   In order to obtain advice from alternative practitioners Americans spent $27 billion dollars. This is a medical expense not covered by insurance companies.
3)   From 1991 to 1997 (only six years), vitamin supplementation increased 130% and herbal therapy increased 380%.
4)   69% of Americans employ some form of alternative medicine.

Current medical schools and most health insurance programs do not believe in alternative health care. Grass root change is occurring at the consumer level. Eventually the change will impact education and health coverage. And mercury amalgams will be part of the change that takes place.

Ben Franklin wrote, "You will observe with concern how long a useful truth may be known and exists, before it is generally received and practiced on". A better statement could not be written today regarding the dangers of mercury amalgams.

Remember the four practical pieces of advice for obtaining good health:

.. DON'T BELIEVE TRADITIONAL MD'S REGARDING MERCURY. They are wrong.
.. DETOXIFYING FROM MERCURY IS A PROCESS, NOT AN EVENT. It takes time, in some cases years.
.. LEARN EVERYTHING YOU CAN FROM THIS BOOK AND OTHER SOURCES OF INFORMATION. Become an expert.
.. DON'T GIVE UP. Stay with the process of detoxification. You will see improvement eventually.

CHAPTER 5

Pride Only Breeds Quarrels But Wisdom Is Found In Those Who Take Advice

SYMPTOMS OF MERCURY TOXICITY

Based on numerous research studies, we know a plethora of symptoms, illnesses and diseases that result from mercury amalgams. It is disappointing, however, that most people only look at mercury toxicity after traditional doctors have given up on them. In my case it took seven years to determine that I was sick, and the allopathic doctors were wrong. My hope is that we can shorten this learning curve to a few weeks, maybe even a few months. If we do this I know that everyone's recovery would be more rapid than it is today based on such a protracted period to diagnosis the illness. Traditionally most people have seen many doctors over many years before they discover that mercury might be the cause of their illness. In reality, "doc shopping" might be the best indicator of mercury toxicity. The patient knows something is wrong but no medical doctor has been able to diagnose the problem. The ultimate solution for the allopathic physician is to send the patient to a shrink.

Interestingly, even the ADA acknowledges that a percentage of people react to mercury amalgams. The ADA states some people have an "allergy" to mercury vapor. The ADA suggests this percentage is very small. Nevertheless, the symptoms associated with this "allergy" are also many of the same symptoms that are identified in this section. So under this scenario people can also have an allergy to arsenic, lead and plutonium. Since when is a toxic element an allergen? It is a poison and people react to poison.

This acknowledgment by the ADA is a double edge sword. At least they admit some people have medical problems associated with mercury amalgams. On the other hand, they believe this problem exists in very few individuals. In other words, a few people get sick from a toxic element but 99.99% of the people with mercury amalgams have no ill effects from inhaling the most toxic non-radioactive element in our universe. Who would believe or even follow that logic? Some day they will have to admit

49

this tragic mistake that resulted in deaths and compromised numerous life styles.

One of the most pressing problems for most mercury toxic people is that from a visual perspective, most look healthy. Beneath this exterior shield their immune system is being compromised and numerous symptoms present themselves that drastically affect everyday life.

This section will be divided into two sections: symptoms that are often present, and symptoms that sometimes accompany mercury poisoning. The reason so many symptoms exist is that mercury has access to every cell in your body.

Mercury is a heavy metal due to the atomic weight of the element. Mercury, as well as other heavy metals such as lead, aluminum, and cadmium, has the ability to displace many of the lighter essential elements. Thus mercury has the ability to replace zinc, magnesium, and other healthy elements in our body.

In addition, mercury is a cytotoxin. A cytotoxin is a toxin poisonous to every living cell it contacts. Mercury has a strong affinity for the sulfur/hydrogen combination that is plentiful in our body. The sulfur/hydrogen combination is referred to as SH, thiol, or sulfhydryl. Each of these references is referred to throughout the book; they are synonymous. When one element has an affinity to another element or combination they can replace that element at binding sites. In addition, the stronger the attraction the harder it is to get the unwanted element to separate. The SH combination is very common in our body. The S represents sulfur and the H hydrogen. The combination occurs frequently in all the sulfur based amino acids, particularly glutathione (GSH). Glutathione is both an amino acid and an antioxidant. Glutathione is present in all cells. When mercury alters the SH molecule in glutathione it alters a critical substance in our body. Glutathione is a primary detoxifying amino acid. It is critical to not only have an ample supply of GSH but also non-compromised GSH.

Amino acids are the building blocks of proteins, and the precursors to cells, hormones and enzymes. When mercury compromises a SH molecule it disrupts the entire process. The cell, hormone, and enzyme no longer function normally. Mercury, a cytotoxin, has poisoned the process.

The ubiquitous nature of the SH molecules in our body poses multiple problems when mercury is present. It affects every cell and organ that requires SH combinations. The initial problem is to eliminate the source of the contamination of the SH protein, the source of the cytotoxin must be eliminated - the mercury amalgam. Next, and the most difficult, is to separate the mercury which is residing on the SH molecule, and finally provide the array of nutrients necessary to reestablish a proper functioning molecule. The latter typically requires a variety of amino acids and vitamins that are synergistic to those specific amino acids.

Once mercury binds to a cell, the cell is poisoned. Since mercury has access to every cell, it is easy to understand the myriad of symptoms that appear.

HERE IS A LIST OF SYMPTOMS THAT ARE OFTEN PRESENT IN THE MERCURY TOXIC INDIVIDUAL:

- mercury fillings, often more than 5 amalgams and usually 10 plus
- a metallic taste in the mouth
- frequent urination during the day, as well as at night.
- short term memory lapses
- fatigue
- irritability and/or periods of depression
- cold hands or feet even in warm weather and a low basal temperature
- heat intolerance and inability to sweat, this is particularly true in females
- headaches
- unexplained gasto-intestinal problems
- anxiety

SYMPTOMS THAT SOMETIMES ACCOMPANY MERCURY TOXICITY:

Symptoms in the mouth

- o bleeding gums in spite of constant flossing
- o general discomfort in the mouth
- o oral galvanization
- o excessive cavities in spite of good dental care
- o root canals

Symptoms in the intestinal tract:

- constipation
- diarrhea
- colitis
- gas
- burping
- food allergies
- hemorrhoids

Symptoms in the psychological area:

- nervousness
- retreat from people situations
- loss of confidence or self esteem
- anger
- temper tantrums
- insomnia
- irritability
- lack of tolerance
- suicide desires
- paranoid feelings
- overactive emotional state
- social withdrawal

Symptoms in other areas:

- changes in blood pressure
- changes in pulse
- dizziness
- changes in heartbeat, or chest pain
- ringing in ears
- asthma
- hay fever
- joint pains, including back, neck, knees etc
- persistent cough
- changes in appetite
- weight loss or weight gain
- chemical sensitivities

- ➢ fibromyalgia
- ➢ elevated cholesterol
- ➢ infections
- ➢ thyroid dysfunction
- ➢ blood sugar problems, diabetes or hypoglycemia
- ➢ hair loss or graying
- ➢ hormone problems
- ➢ hearing loss
- ➢ speech disorders
- ➢ cataracts
- ➢ tremors

Unlike the flu, mercury poisoning is a slow process. It starts with a few symptoms. It continues its assault, and more and more organs are affected. No place is safe from the ravages of mercury vapor and the subsequent forms of mercury poisoning. It is believed that some heart attacks are caused by mercury based on the negative impact mercury has on magnesium. Specifically, mercury can replace magnesium in your tissue and cells and magnesium is an essential product that your heart needs to function properly. Additionally, it is fair to say that kidney and liver impairments are frequently caused by mercury.

I do not want to open up the entire issue of cancer, but if you believe that cancer proliferates when portions of the immune system break down – what does a better job of negatively impacting the immune system than mercury? Is it possible that mercury toxicity is the precursor to many cancers? Could the following cycle actually occur? Mercury is present in your system. Your immune system tries to rid itself of this toxin. Your immune system slowly loses the battle and mercury can now take advantage of a suppressed immune system.

The following is more than just a hypothetical scenario. Mercury enters a cell, and affects the DNA. DNA is a complex maze of amino acids attached by threads. The threads are strands. When the DNA is broken a single strand break occurs. This malfunction continues in each generation of cell reproduction. DNA is replicating itself albeit in an altered and unhealthy state. Mercury is one cause of a potential break; X-rays are another example of DNA alteration. The result of any single strand break is carcinogenic. This is the reason X-rays are considered carcinogenic. The repair process for strand breaks are reductase enzymes. Thus concluding mercury is a potential cancer cause is not a huge scientific leap. Some medical doctors, and even medical clinics, state unequivocally that every cancer patient is mercury toxic. This is a bold statement and without research to support it today, but definitely something for each of us to ponder. I wonder if the American Cancer Society is prepared to analyze this statement. Based on the amount of money that is raised for research, I think it would be worthwhile to allocate a few bucks to see if this statement has merit. And when did cancer become such a health problem? The answer – about the same time we started using mercury amalgams indiscriminately.

To summarize, mercury attacks individuals differently. Symptoms that are described in this chapter exhibit themselves slowly over time, multiply and eventually unfold as some form of autoimmune disease, cancer, heart disease or any number of conditions not generally associated with mercury.

The four important attributes to recovery are

. . DON'T BELIEVE TRADITIONAL MD's REGARDING MERCURY. They are wrong.
. . DETOXIFYING FROM MERCURY IS A PROCESS, NOT AN EVENT. It takes time, in some cases years.
. . LEARN EVERYTHING YOU CAN FROM THIS AND OTHER SOURCES OF INFORMATION. Become an expert.
. . DON'T GIVE UP. Stay with the process of detoxification. You will see improvement eventually.

CHAPTER 6

Instruct A Wise Man And He Will Be Wiser Still; Teach A Righteous Man And He Will Add To His Leaving

OK, MAYBE I'M MERCURY TOXIC ... WHAT DO I DO NEXT?

Mercury compromises every immune system. If an immune system is compromised, then the opportunity for disease increases. In order to understand the slow poison that amalgams create look at the simple task of breathing. We take about 17000 breaths a day. With each breath we inhale a microdose of mercury from our amalgams. It takes on average 60 days to eliminate 50% of the inhaled mercury. Thus look at the progression;

Day 1 – 1 part mercury inhaled, 0 parts eliminated.
Day 2 – 1 part mercury inhaled, cumulative 2 parts inhaled, 0 parts eliminated
Day 61 – 61 parts mercury inhaled, .5 parts eliminated, 60.5 parts accumulated.
Day 360 – 360 parts mercury inhaled, 50 parts eliminated, 210 parts accumulated.

Ten, 20, or 50 years of mercury vapor is a death sentence. The only question is which death sentence, which your system is going to lose the battle to – cancer, MS, heart disease, Alzheimer's, etc.

Any section of any book on testing for mercury suggests that criteria used to determine mercury toxicity is changing rapidly and it is best to keep apprised of new technology and new methodologies to determine potential mercury levels. Let me start by telling you what *not* to do. Do not go to your internist and tell him/her that you read a book on mercury amalgams and you think this is the cause of your poor health. Remember, most medical doctors have been trained and brainwashed to believe that mercury in your mouth is just fine. Not only will your internist tell you that you are wrong but he also will say that you are crazy and that you need to stop looking for solutions so far off main street. In addition, do not pose this same question to your dentist. They have the same training, and same beliefs. Basically this group of traditional practitioners will not help you. They may affect your desire to pursue a solution. A very appropriate statement applies to both doctors and uninformed patients: "It's not what you don't know that kills you – it's what you do know that isn't correct that kills you." The real danger is doctors and dentists, and most health care consumers believe that mercury is benign in their dental fillings. So what should a health care consumer do if they believe mercury vapor from amalgams are affecting their health?

First of all, try and find a clinic in your area that has some specialty in mercury or environmental illness. Next look to see if there are any medical doctors that specialize in mercury toxicity. Unless you are in a big city, this might be a challenge. Many times if neither of these avenues is successful a naturopathic physician might be helpful. However, since one of the ways to determine if you are truly mercury toxic is a DMPS challenge (and only MDs and DOs can administer this test), it would be better for everyone to work with a medical doctor, even if that means traveling some distance. There are a couple of places to look for a doctor. Write to DAMS (Dental Amalgam Mercury Syndrome), Post Office Box 7249, Minneapolis MN 55407-0249. DAMS produces a periodic newsletter that is a great resource. They also have a list of doctors and dentists who work with mercury toxic patients. Another valuable source of information is "Dental and Health Facts, Foundation for Toxic Free Dentistry," P.O. Box 608010, Orlando Florida 32860-8010. This group provides information, a newsletter and is also very helpful. Also the web sites referenced earlier in the book might be helpful.

In order to determine if you are mercury toxic, there are a number of different methodologies to choose from. The first option is to look inside your mouth. Do you have "a lot" of amalgams? How many amalgam surfaces do you have? If the answer is "a lot" you may have already diagnosed the problem. I guarantee if the answer is "yes" to this question, if it is not the cause of your illness, then it is at the very least adding to your health burden. If you are ill with many of the symptoms suggested earlier and you have a mouthful of mercury amalgams, then remove them. Mercury might not be the cause, but it is certainly compromising good health.

Assuming you want confirmation of the inspection you made of your mouth, you should have a hair analysis done. A hair analysis measures the physiological or nutrient metabolism at the cellular level. This test shows if you are secreting mercury through your scalp and into your hair. A reading above the norm is indicative of mercury poisoning. However, a normal reading does not mean you are mercury free. It might mean that you are storing mercury and simply not releasing it. Some researchers believe only methylmercury is indicated in a hair analysis. Regardless, if the mercury reading is high, then mercury is a problem. However, the reading does not necessarily correlate with the body burden. In other words, if the hair analysis shows only a slightly elevated level that does not mean you are only slightly toxic. You could be acutely toxic. Some researchers believe hair mercury only applies to the brain burden. Thus according to this group, very little measured mercury in the hair means almost nothing when it comes to determining mercury toxicity in non-brain organs.

A hair analysis is also helpful in determining other heavy metals that might be a problem, as well as and mineral imbalances and deficiencies. Often vitamin and mineral levels determine toxicity even if the metals are stored and not being released. The test is about $75.00 and is a great place to start. Allopathic doctors initially viewed hair analysis with skepticism; however, almost all now agree that hair provides an excellent analysis of certain heavy metals, these include: mercury, lead, aluminum, cadmium, tin, nickel, and arsenic.

If the hair analysis does not indicate elevated mercury, there are other indicators in the hair analysis that are very suggestive of mercury toxicity. Often mercury is not excreted in the hair and thus, since it does not show up as elevated in the hair analysis, it is often times dismissed as a possible problem. This is a huge mistake. In all probability the person has a very slow metabolic rate and thus mercury remains sequestered in tissue and various organs. This suggests detoxifying from mercury will be a more prolonged process. The simple fact that it is not being excreted is the reason that it is not elevated. But other mineral readings in a hair analysis are often times just as accurate in predicting a mercury problem.

1. Low zinc and/or high copper. This often times exists since zinc is competing with mercury at binding sites. If mercury wins, and it always does, zinc will be low. If zinc is low the antagonist mineral, copper will be elevated and this will only add to your problems. This has a particularly negative effect on metallothioneins. These are intercellular proteins that serve as storage complexes for zinc and

copper. However they have a strong affinity for all heavy metals, especially mercury. Metallothioneins also are high in cysteine, which is a sulfur-based amino acid.

2. <u>Low sodium and/or low potassium</u>. Sodium is excreted in your urine as your body attempts to rid tissue of mercury, often excessively. Sodium and potassium work synergistically and if one is low the other is often low as well.

3. <u>Low magnesium</u>. Another important mineral that is often replaced by mercury. Low magnesium is often associated with high mercury levels. Mercury competes with magnesium on a molecule for molecule basis. Mercury is heavier but it is essentially the same size electrically. When mercury replaces magnesium a host of problems occur including muscular skeletal and intestinal issues. Magnesium is critical for heart health. If you have an anxiety problem, then it can probable that magnesium is low. Magnesium is a natural sedative.

4. <u>Low sulfur</u>. Sulfur is a carrier to help mercury leave the body. When sulfur is low it signals excessive usage.

5. <u>Elevated heavy metals including lead, aluminum, silver, tin, and nickel</u>. Silver, tin, and nickel are often used in an amalgam.

6. <u>Low lithium</u>.

7. <u>Elevated calcium</u>. This is the non-biological form of calcium. This form interferes with zinc, magnesium, and manganese absorption. This in conjunction with low magnesium, often suggest blood sugar problems.

8. <u>Low phosphorus</u>. Phosphorus is often lost, via the kidney, while trying to eliminate mercury. Frequent urination is a typical sign of mercury toxicity and this frequently eliminates important minerals, including phosphorous.

The hair analysis provides absolute numbers for a variety of toxic heavy metals and healthy metals. A few ratios might also suggest a mercury problem:

1. Zinc/Mercury should be 200:1 or higher
2. Selenium/Mercury should be 1:1 or higher
3. Sulfur/Mercury should be 28000:1 or higher

If mercury is not demonstrating itself in the heavy metal portion of the hair analysis, the above eight indicators and three ratios are important in diagnosing possible mercury problems. If mercury is demonstrating itself, then many of the above will also exist.

Another indicator is your cholesterol level. Studies indicate high TSC in mercury toxic people. The theory is that cholesterol is actually acting as an antioxidant, protecting the body from mercury. If your diet is excellent, you exercise regularly, and cannot lower your TSC, mercury might be the reason. Some doctors believe LDL is an indicator of mercury problems; high LDL is considered by many a mercury marker. Be careful of drugs that guarantee to lower TSC. Studies indicate when TSC is lowered suddenly there is an increased incidence of murder, suicide, and other types of fatalities. Elevated TSH may also indicate a congested liver.

Basal temperature first thing in the morning represents thyroid function. Typically a low temperature indicates a thyroid problem. The traditional approach is to confirm a malfunctioning thyroid with a blood test and prescribe a thyroid drug. However, the problem might be mercury. The thyroid is located very close to teeth and thus mercury amalgams. Mercury has a strong affinity for iodine, a primary component of the thyroid. Thus the proximity and attraction for iodine makes the thyroid an easy place for mercury to park. To test this theory, take your temperature under your arm first thing in the morning. If it is below 97.8 degrees suspect mercury. The conversion of T4 to T3 requires certain enzymes and cofactors, and mercury typically compromises this conversion and the result is a low temperature.

The Coors Study mentioned previously measured prophyrins released in the urine as an indicator. This is a good test, but make sure the laboratory in your area is capable of producing valid test results. The test is expensive and if other tests suggest mercury is the problem it may not be necessary to use this particular test.

Some doctors have meters that determine the electrical reading from your mercury amalgams fillings. If you are fortunate to find a doctor that has this equipment, you can determine if you are releasing mercury vapor and which teeth are the most toxic. It is an easy test and another great indicator.

A recent study indicates that a venous blood gas test is an excellent tool for analyzing a potential mercury problem. One of the results of mercury toxicity is a compromised venous blood gas. This test measures the oxygen saturation of your blood; the norm is 80-85%. If you have a reading that is less than this, mercury is a likely reason. Even your internist will agree that if this result is low, then something is wrong. He may not agree with mercury as the cause but he should at least have to scratch his head. In my case, my venous blood gas was 28%. I was sick and this supported my contention. It was the only test, of all the tests that I took, and these tests included CBC, thyroid functions, adrenal panels, etc., which was not within normal ranges. In a small sample of mercury patients at a holistic doctor's office in the Pacific Northwest, every single person had an oxygen test result, based on a venous blood gas test, significantly below the normal range. This is not a perfect predictor based on sample size, but try it and see what your results are. This test must be done at a hospital since the blood must be analyzed very quickly after it is drawn. The prescription from your doctor must be specific so the correct test is done. The prescription should read:

> Venous (NOT arterial) blood gas for OXYHEMOGLOBIN SATURATION
> Co-Oximeter is OK
> Pulse Oximeter is NOT acceptable

This test also measures CO_2 in the blood and if oxygen is low CO_2 were probably be high.

Before we go any further, let's review blood. Blood is comprised of plasma, red blood cells, white blood cells, platelets, proteins and gases. There are other components of blood, but the above are our primary concern. Also, remember that mercury has a strong affinity for sulfur. The function of red blood cells is to transport oxygen throughout the body. Mercury attaches itself to sulfur groups found on red blood cells. Mercury, as well as other metals, replaces oxygen at binding sights on the red blood cell. The result of this action is fatigue. Oxygen is removed and mercury has replaced it.

Do not despair when you get the results of your venous blood gas test. Through various protocols you can reverse this process and get oxygen back into your hemoglobin molecules and rid yourself of the effects of mercury. It is important to monitor your oxygen readings periodically. This test is expensive and an option that can be used is to have a qualified person visually examine the color of your blood. If your blood is very dark that means there is less oxygen content. The lighter the color means there is greater oxygen content. Once mercury binds to the SH group on the hemoglobin molecule it has replaced a site designed for oxygen. Each hemoglobin molecule has four such sites. Each red blood cell has 300 molecules. If oxygen is on all of them venous is 100%. As each molecule is compromised, mercury has replaced oxygen, symptoms occur. The most common problem is fatigue.

Another test is an adrenal panel. This measures the stress that adrenal function is experiencing. There are two possible results: either elevated cortisol production, or reduced production. Case one is probably early in the toxicity process. The adrenals are working overtime to combat mercury. Case two is probably late in the process. You have temporarily lost the battle, adrenal function is low, and fatigue is a major symptom. In the latter case it is important to recharge the adrenals and increase the output of cortisol. This helps regain the sense of well-being. A discussion of adrenal support will be elaborated on later in the book.

A CBC yields indicators of mercury toxicity. However most will be within the range that the laboratory establishes. Suspect mercury problems if WBC, monocytes, basophils, and platelets are at the high end of the acceptable range. In addition lymphocytes and eosinophils will be at the low end of the range.

As a frame of reference, the results of the above tests/indicators for me were the following:

- Hair analysis: high mercury, low zinc, seriously elevated copper, low magnesium, sodium, potassium, sulfur, lithium, chromium, and elevated calcium

- Mercury electrical reader was not available to me.

- Venous oxygen reading of 29 (norm 80), CO_2 marginally elevated from norm.

- TSC 250, high LDL

- A basal temperature 95.4 degrees, this suggests a seriously malfunctioning thyroid. The thyroid is a master gland and controls many functions of the endocrine system.

- The prophyrin test not available at the time I was trying to diagnose mercury.

- An adrenal panel was taken after mercury was already diagnosed. Cortisol levels were significantly below standard at all four stages of testing.

- WBC and platelets were severely elevated.

Individually each test was a strong indicator; collectively they confirmed mercury was a major problem.

My suggestion is to use the above criteria to determine if you are mercury toxic. If they are conclusive, get your mercury amalgams removed.

Many doctors administer a DMPS challenge as another indicator of mercury toxicity. If you decide to use this protocol, be very careful, and read this entire section. Using DMPS before all mercury amalgams are removed can be dangerous. It needs to be administered by a medical doctor that understands chelation and the effects of DMPS.

DMPS is a German medication that binds to heavy metals and eliminates the toxin from your body primarily through your kidneys. DMPS is an acid molecule with two free SH groups that binds heavy metals. It is approved in Germany by the BGA (Germany's version of the FDA) for treatment of mercury poisoning. Research indicates this is a reasonably safe medication when administered by someone with knowledge and when used after *all* mercury amalgams have been removed. If you decide to use DMPS prior to amalgam removal (remember this book is advising you not to do this, but some doctors recommend it), the first thing that needs to be checked is your creatine clearance. This determines how efficient your kidneys are working and may determine how much DMPS is administered. Your doctor may give you up to 5 cc's of DMPS in an IV over a 20 minute time frame. Your job over the next six hours is to retain all your urine. Get a couple of containers from your doctor. You may find yourself urinating a lot. During this six-hour collection period you may have a few side effects or none at all. The side effects are the result of mercury being mobilized and *hopefully* eliminated from your system. Return to the doctor with your urine the next day and get a vitamin and mineral IV. This is critical. DMPS not only binds to mercury, but it also binds to other minerals that your body needs, such as chromium, zinc and copper. The

IV replenishes your missing vitamins and minerals. Now you need to wait.

DMPS is one of a number of chelators that are discussed in this book. Chelate comes from the Greek word meaning claw. Chelators are chemicals that hold other chemicals, similar to a claw. Chelators only attract metals, such as mercury, copper, iron, zinc, and chromium. The most important function of a chelator is that it can enter and exit a cell membrane. The goal is that the chelator "grabs" onto mercury and eliminates it using the kidneys or intestines.

Since mercury has a strong affinity for SH combinations, and since this affinity makes that separation difficult, it is therefore critical to use chelators that can break that attraction. DMPS is one chelator that can break mercury from a SH molecule. Remember the half life of mercury? Without using a chelator to expedite the removal of mercury you will not live long enough to eliminate all the mercury that is causing illness and compromising your quality of life. Measuring the mercury in urine after taking DMPS determines how much mercury may be in your system, but most important is how much was excreted.

A few words of caution regarding DMPS are appropriate. Most literature supports the safety of this medication, but there are reports of severe side effects in some individuals. It appears the most drastic side effects are in the individuals who are the most toxic and who use DMPS prior to having all their mercury amalgams removed. If you are deciding whether to try it or not, it is probably a subjective decision based on the outcome of various tests, the knowledge and experience of the doctor, and the amount of risk the patient wants to take. DMPS is a double edge sword. It becomes more and more dangerous as levels of mercury increase. At the same time, this is precisely the individual that needs mercury excretion expedited. The reason for the side effects is that DMPS is excellent at mobilizing mercury. It "stirs it up" vigorously. However, our body is very poor at eliminating all this "stirred up" mercury. When it is not eliminated, it finds new binding sites, often worse than before the original mobilization. Thus, we experience the side effects. It has been reported that side effects are reduced when 25 grams of vitamin C is administered via IV prior to the 20 minute DMPS IV.

As mentioned, many doctors use a DMPS challenge as a toxicity tool in evaluating a patient. Personally I would not recommend this test until all mercury has been removed from a patient's mouth. DMPS actually pulls mercury from mercury amalgams and this rapid excretion from a patient's tooth creates huge amounts of mercury that cannot be eliminated by the patient. It then finds binding sites in various organs in the body. The consequences can be very dangerous. However, some doctors do recommend this test, and as a patient, you need to be aware that it is a tool to determine toxicity albeit with potentially serious consequences.

The difference between a DMPS challenge (a test to measure mercury levels and to determine if mercury toxicity exists) and DMPS as a protocol is that five cc's of DMPS (depending on weight) is usually given to measure toxicity in a challenge. The more DMPS that is used the greater the probability of side effects. The reality is that any amount of DMPS can be used when conducting a challenge or as a protocol to use after the removal of all mercury from the oral cavity. It does not have to be the maximum dosage of 5 cc's. Any amount of DMPS results in mercury being released via the kidneys and into the urine. In order to determine if mercury is a problem, it is not necessary to give the maximum amount of DMPS and potentially create side effects. A nominal amount can produce enough information to be a predictor. If a patient and doctor decide to start with reduced amounts of DMPS, once mercury amalgams have been removed, and DMPS is used frequently it makes sense to slowly increase the amount that is used, assuming no side effects result from the previous dosage. The greater amount of DMPS results in greater excretion of mercury. But build to the maximum dosage slowly if you are concerned with side effects, or if other indicators suggest your mercury burden is high. Some practitioners can test for adverse reactions to DMPS before using it through muscle testing or Electro Dermal screening.

DMSA is another excellent chelator that can be used to measure mercury excretion. DMSA is typically much safer than DMPS but it does not chelate as much mercury as DMPS. However if safety is a concern, and it should be, a DMSA challenge and DMSA as a protocol, can also provide valuable information. Again, I would caution against using DMSA as a toxicity tool. It also pulls mercury from amalgams in a similar fashion to DMPS. Wait and use it after all mercury amalgams have been removed. Often doctors suggest other chelators, particularly EDTA; do not waste your money or your time. The only effective chelators of mercury are DMPS and DMSA.

It typically takes about two weeks to get this test result back. If the test was used to determine toxicity levels to determine whether to get your mercury amalgams removed, use this time to get an appointment with a mercury free dentist. In order to find a mercury free dentist, use your doctor, DAMS, Foundation for Toxic Free Dentistry, the yellow pages, and word of mouth, etc. Typically these dentists are very busy and waiting periods can be 4-6 weeks. Call as many dentists as you can and interview each of them. All qualified dentists will use special precautions when removing mercury. Discuss these protocols with each of them. Find someone you are comfortable with and who will work with you on a timeline that makes sense. Also since this is an expensive proposition many dentists will work with you on a payment plan.

The combined results of the above tests should provide the necessary information to determine if mercury is a problem.

Remember the four critical principals:

.. DON'T BELIEVE TRADITIONAL MD'S REGARDING MERCURY. They are wrong.
.. DETOXIFYING FROM MERCURY IS A PROCESS, NOT AN EVENT. It takes time, in some cases years.
.. LEARN EVERYTHING YOU CAN FROM THIS BOOK AND OTHER SOURCES OF INFORMATION. Become an expert.
.. DON'T GIVE UP. Stay with the process of detoxification. You will see improvement eventually.

CHAPTER 7

FOR WISDOM IS MORE PRECIOUS THAN RUBIES

OK, I'M MERCURY TOXIC! HOW DO I DETOXIFY?

There are multiple steps involved in answering this question. First you need to make an appointment with a dentist. Second you need to determine a medical protocol to get the mercury out of your system and this will include some type of chelator, DMPS or DMSA, as well as a process for getting vitamins and minerals back into your body. Remember, your hair analysis probably showed mineral deficiencies that need to be balanced as the mercury is removed.

Since your dental fillings have made you sick, it makes sense to get your mercury amalgams removed as quickly as possible. Sort of correct. At this point, all you know is that mercury amalgams make you sick, but did you know that some composites also contain metals that can cause problems for an already compromised immune system? In order to avoid going through this process twice, get a compatibility test done on the composite alternatives that are available.   Jess Clifford in Colorado Springs (719-550-0008) can do a blood test on not only the materials that will be used in filling your cavities but also on cements etc. By having this test done you will guarantee that the materials being used in your mouth will not cause problems.   Do this ... it may sound like an unnecessary process but I had all my mercury removed only to find out the composite used contained different incompatible metals, and I had to redo the process all over again. This is not fun. It is very expensive, time consuming, and delays good health unnecessarily. Your doctor will be able to administer the compatibility test and send the blood sample for analysis.

Once you have decided on the type of dental material you want to use its important that your dentist use some common protocols. First, insist that he use a rubber dam. This will insure that you do not swallow or inhale any mercury or mercury vapor during the removal procedure. Also it is important that some highly toxic individuals breathe oxygen during the procedure. In addition during your interview process, you should insure the dentist office has an excellent ventilation system.

Most often it will take four or five appointments for the dentist to accomplish the task of getting all the mercury out of your mouth. If the dentist can do more than one quadrant at a time then you can expedite the process. Usually a fifth appointment is necessary to fit any crowns that are made while working on the final quadrant. Be sure crowns are not metallic in any fashion. Mercury disables cells, nickel which is used in 85% of all crowns turn cells malignant. Nickel has been a known carcinogen for 50 years. But it is still used in crowns, braces and bridges.

Unfortunately, having the mercury removed is not like having your appendix out. If you have an inflamed appendix removed, usually within a few weeks you are starting to function again normally. The removal of mercury amalgams deals with the source of your illness. Obviously very important but the real work comes trying to remove all the mercury that has found a home in your various organs. The body burden of mercury is similar to rain collecting in a barrel. It fills gradually, and we adjust at low levels of toxicity. But as the barrel fills and eventually overflows we experience toxic overload. Our natural detoxification mechanisms fail and our list of symptoms grow. Symptoms turn into diseases. The secret is to empty the rain barrel so that toxic inflow can be easily managed by our detoxification systems.

I guarantee that at a minimum if you have mercury amalgams it is compromising your brain, thyroid, kidneys, liver, gastro system, and immune system. And remember from your venous blood gas test we already know the oxygen content of your blood has been compromised. Additionally, mercury has replaced magnesium, and zinc in your body. We need to remove the mercury so we can let normal, healthy and important vitamins and minerals take the place of mercury and do their job. That job is insuring your good health. OK, so how do I begin?

A GOOD NIGHTS SLEEP

Detoxification is the process of eliminating toxins from your body. Prior to starting any intense detoxification process, it is necessary to address foundations. Additionally, it is important to understand detoxification is a parasympathetic function. It is more active at rest and at night. A good night's sleep is as important as anything that you can do to prepare your body to eliminate toxins. The process of detoxification frees cellular energy that was being compromised by xenobiotics (toxins) and produces a sense of well being. In order to insure 8 hours of sleep per night avoid eating sugar, consuming caffeine, dealing with confrontation and stress, watching TV and worrying or obsessing about life's trivia. Sleep is enhanced by soaking in a chlorine free hot tub, having pleasant conversations, reading a good book, meditating or going for a short walk. The most important foundation to address in addition to rest is the food you eat.

NUTRITION, NUTRITION, NUTRITION

The process of regaining your health will depend on a number of changes and commitments to protocols that you never imagined. The first change that must be made is adhering to a healthy diet. I guarantee your diet is not healthy, and that is based on choices you make in your daily eating habits, and some of your decisions are because of massive marketing done by drug companies and fast food chains.

A recent study conducted by the National Cancer Institute discovered that only 9% of Americans eat 5 servings of fruits or vegetables per day. One in nine surveyed did not eat any fruits and vegetables daily. Different surveys have discovered that almost 50% of every food dollar is spent away from the home, and the average American consumes approximately 50 pounds of high fructose corn syrup per year, drinks more soft drinks than water, and spends over $75 billion on fast food and over $50 billion on soft drinks. If you are part of the above statistics you need to undergo dramatic life style changes. The foundation of good health is good nutrition. The following are a few important guidelines in order to recover from disease, chronic health problems, and improve your quality of life.

1. **Drink at least 64 oz. of water every day.** Water is the most important change you can make to your nutrition program. Water is crucial for hydrating cells and membranes, and eliminating waste products. A shortage of water is the cause of a whole host of health problems, including joint pain, constipation, headaches, fatigue, and allergies. Avoid water that has been contaminated with chlorine, and fluoride. Use filtered water or distilled water. Don't worry if you drink more than 64 oz a day, this is the minimum requirement.

2. **Eat lots of vegetables.** A guideline is at least 50% of all the food you eat every day should be vegetables. They provide an excellent source of vitamins and minerals, which is important in detoxification. It is OK to eat some fruit but do

not substitute fruit for vegetables. Vegetables that are rich in color are the best. Potatoes do not count as a source of vegetables. It will be necessary to eat vegetables that you have not tried before, use them in different ways and in different combinations. It will improve your energy, mental clarity and help eliminate toxins. Invest in a good cookbook, and eat only organic if possible.

3. **Avoid all hydrogenated oils.** Hydrogenated oil is the food industry's method of turning liquid oil into fat. This prolongs the shelf life of the processed foods and increases the profitability of the food producer. Hydrogenated oil produces trans fats, which have been linked to the following health problems: cancer, heart disease, increased levels of cholesterol, joint pain, arthritis, immune system malfunction, depression and fatigue. Simply put, hydrogenated oils are not healthy in any fashion; they are convenient. This is not to suggest that all fats are bad for you; some are very healthy and should be part of an everyday diet; coconut oil, flaxseed oil, olive oil, and oils that come from organic (not roasted) nuts. Avoid all foods that are fried, all chips, crackers, cereals and breads that contain hydrogenated oil. In addition read labels carefully on salad dressings and mayonnaise. Butter is a good fat and margarine contains trans fats. A Harvard study of 90,000 nurses showed margarine usage increased the probability of heart disease by 50%.

4. **Eliminate sugar of all types.** In 1750 the average consumption of sugar in England was 7 pounds per year per adult. Today, an average American consumes over 120 pounds of refined sugar per year. Sugar consumption increases insulin and adrenal hormone production and causes the body to excrete important minerals. The effect of this chain reaction is the following; your body needs additional vitamins, particularly all the B's and C. Yeast increases in the bowel producing toxins and reducing the good bacteria necessary for proper digestion. Massive changes in blood sugar levels occur, and inflammation increases. If it is impossible to eliminate sugar completely try stevia, agave, or other natural substitutes. It may be necessary to give up sugar cold turkey. It is an addiction that demands willpower.

5. **Eliminate refined carbohydrates.** Most Americans get over 50% of their calories from refined carbohydrates. These are

grains that have had their fiber and vitamins removed. All that is left is starch. Refined carbohydrates fill you up, without vitamin and mineral enrichment and cause stress on your digestive system, and your endocrine system. In many ways sugar and refined carbohydrates is the same product. They provide no nutritional value, and cause harm to all of the regulatory functions in your body. Everything that does not have the words whole grain is refined. Do not eat white rice; instead enjoy the nutrition of brown rice.

6. **Eliminate all chemical additives.** The average American consumes and processes through their digestive system 10 pounds of chemicals every year in their food and beverages. One of largest chemical consumed is aspartame. This has been linked to cancer, headaches, depression and memory loss. Instead drink water with an organic lemon.

7. **Take your time eating. Never miss a meal. Be sure to consume some protein.** Chew until your food is soft and almost in a liquid state. The extra time chewing activates enzymes in your saliva and improves digestion. If you miss a meal your metabolism will decrease and the result is fatigue. Enjoy snacks everyday. Some vegetables, a piece of fruit or nuts. This helps regulate blood sugar. Protein is the building block of all amino acids and is critical for a healthy existence. Everyone should consume 4-6 oz. of organic protein at each of their primary meals. All meats should be nitrate free. Protein drinks are popular snacks and they are fine as long as they do not contain soy. The best are non denatured whey drinks or goat protein. In addition, eat eggs. Eggs are a complete protein source, they contain every amino acid, enjoy one of the only whole foods. Chose eggs that organic, free range, fertile, and enhanced. Enhanced means the hens have been fed an enriched diet that improves their nutritional value. Don't limit yourself to chicken eggs, try duck eggs.

8. **Eliminate caffeine.** Caffeine poses numerous problems. Since caffeine is a foreign substance it is the livers job to eliminate it. The last thing your liver needs is another detoxification responsibility. In addition caffeine increases blood pressure, contributes to adrenal exhaustion, elevates cortisol and lowers DHEA, disrupts sleep, adversely affects the immune system, contributes to magnesium deficiencies, impairs digestion and creates hormonal imbalances. If all that

is not a problem, caffeine is addictive. If you are hooked on caffeine slowly eliminate all caffeine products. Do not go cold turkey. Your body will react to the sudden elimination of caffeine. Its addictive properties are a marketing plus for companies that promote the product.

THE VALUE OF STOMACH ACID

Most readers of this book read stomach acid and their immediate reaction is negative. We are bombarded with commercials that state the horrible consequences of stomach acid and remedies that are readily available from drug companies. In one large chain, there were 22 different products to reduce the effects of stomach acid. Did you know that stomach acid is as crucial for your health as oxygen, sulfur and water? Did you know that reducing your stomach acid level causes disease and illness? Did you know that on the rare occasion that acid indigestion occurs a digestive enzyme works better than advertised remedies without the negative impact?

The entire digestive system is regulated by a variety of pH levels. It all starts with adequate stomach acid (HCL). If you have too much HCL you feel a burning, commonly referred to as acid indigestion, and if you have to little you feel absolutely nothing. However, you cannot absorb vitamins and minerals or amino acids. The ability to nourish your body regardless of how well you eat is impossible.

Inadequate amounts of stomach acid are acknowledged as a problem; it is called hypochlorhydria. However, mainstream medicine does not test for it, and for the most part does not recognize the implications of the problem. When the pH of the stomach is not optimal, the pH in the rest of the digestive process will also be off. Stomach acid begins to secrete on the simple act of chewing, and impacts all hormones, vitamins, minerals, proteins, fats, amino acids, sugars, oils and carbohydrates. A few reasons why a person can have low stomach acid:

1. Heavy metal toxicity
2. Infections
3. A malfunctioning liver, due to toxicity from drugs, chemicals and metals
4. Disease
5. Mineral imbalance, often caused by heavy metals

6. Excessive use of antacids
7. A significant toxic exposure
8. Stress, both physical and emotional – exhausted adrenals
9. Low levels of zinc. Typically low zinc will predict low stomach acid.

Most mercury toxic individuals are so concerned with getting the mercury out that they forget to support a digestive system that allows for efficient detoxification. It is impossible to detoxify completely without adequate stomach acid levels. In many ways, it is a vicious cycle; mercury reduces stomach acid due to a number of metabolically compromised functions; this makes it difficult to eliminate the toxins since stomach acid is inadequate to facilitate excretions, and thus mercury will continue to increase and cause more and more symptoms. But this piece of the puzzle is easy to fix, simply replace the lost HCL. It is easy and very inexpensive. But before discussing the dosage and the methodology, what symptoms occur due to inadequate stomach acid? The list is lengthy.

Two very common symptoms are hypoglycemia and hypothyroidism. Low blood sugar is a result of the inability to digest protein. Over 50% of digested protein is converted to glucose. If we are not digesting protein we are robbing our body of valuable glucose. In addition, there are deficiencies in magnesium, chromium, and zinc. These minerals are all necessary to maintain proper levels of blood sugar. Glucose is fuel. With reduced levels we get traditional symptoms: hunger, faintness, dizziness, headache and fatigue.

The thyroid is often called the master gland. It impacts the adrenals, liver function, and hormones. The thyroid requires a number of vitamins and minerals to function properly. It demands all the B vitamins and all the minerals mentioned above. The B vitamins are important for a number of reasons, not the least of which is that they are necessary for the production of enzymes. And the proper production of healthy enzymes is required for every bodily function; they keep us alive. Thus when we are unable to assimilate the B vitamins, along with the minerals; iodine, zinc, selenium, magnesium, molybdenum, and various amino acids, and especially tyrosine our thyroid begins malfunctioning. In addition, the thyroid, due to its proximity to mercury vapor from our dental amalgam, will attract mercury and cause even more problems. A common symptom of thyroid problems is either low body temperature or feeling hot in only moderate temperatures.

Other problems associated with low HCL are: headaches, B12 deficiency, high blood pressure, stroke, elevated cholesterol, and/or homocysteine levels, intestinal bacteria, dysbiosis, (HCL is the best antibacterial available to kill bugs and bacteria residing in the intestines), autism, most autoimmune diseases, congested liver, pancreatitis, kidney stones, muscular aches and pains, bone spurs, osteoporosis, and additional heavy metal toxicity particularly cadmium and aluminum. Thus low HCL will have a major impact if it is not addressed immediately, and will make the efficiency of any protocols for detoxification impossible if adequate levels of HCL are not produced.

Low levels of HCL makes it impossible to assimilate the B vitamins and this means that many enzymes will not work in the critical phase 1 and phase 2 detoxification pathways. In addition low HCL leads to low levels of magnesium and this critical mineral has a plethora of functions in virtually every organ in the human body.

Solving stomach acid problems is the easiest part of the detoxification process. If you suspect HCL problems, buy a bottle of HCL with pepsin and take one capsule at one of your main meals. If you feel burning or warmth in your stomach, stop and drink some water or eat additional food; the sensation will disappear. If the problem occurs with one capsule, discontinue the experiment and inform your doctor. However, if you have no discomfort, continue adding capsules of HCL at each main meal. For example if you are up to five capsules take one when you are 1/5th through your meal, and add a capsule at each 1/5th interval. Continue this until you get the feeling of warmth in your stomach. Your dosage is one capsule less than that amount. At snacks, determine your dosage in the same fashion. It is possible for a person to be taking up a large number of capsules at each meal. Keep increasing until you reach the proper dosage. One word of caution; it is possible that if you took large amount of antacids at some point that you have destroyed the sensitivity in your stomach and you never feel the sensation of warmth in your stomach regardless of the amount of HCL you consume. Be very careful in this situation and work with a doctor to determine responsible and therapeutic amounts of HCL. If you require large amounts of HCL, include non-flush macin with each meal; the dosage should be at least 100 mgs per meal. At the end of each meal take a pancreatic enzyme. In all probability your pancreas is compromised so nourish your digestive process with this enzyme. It may take months before you start to feel better but you will.

During this period avoid fasting and drink plenty of water. Between meals take bromelain. This is a great digestive enzyme made from pineapple. Depending on how compromised your digestive system you may find yourself taking lots of HCL everyday, three meals plus snacks. But do it. In addition, be sure to take your supplements with meals when there is plenty of HCL in your system to provide adequate absorption. Adequate stomach acid is mandatory in order to digest and absorb food and supplements.

A CHELATOR TO REMOVE THE MERCURY

DMPS is a good chelator for some people and should be given by a trained medical doctor. This is the fastest way to remove mercury. However, as mentioned previously, under no circumstances should you commence DMPS until all your dental work is completed. It is not the only way, as we will discuss, but a very efficient way to remove mercury assuming DMPS can be tolerated. DMPS can be given as frequently as every week. Frequency will be determined by your doctor and is based on dosage, symptoms, and reaction. DMPS is such a strong chelator one risk is to do it too infrequently. If it is not administered often DMPS disrupts more mercury than you can eliminate and re deposits it in other organs. The redeposit process can be worse than the original symptoms. So administer any chelator frequently, and keep the mercury mobilized and constantly in the process of elimination. The dosage of DMPS varies by weight and risk. It is best to start with a very low dosage and gradually increase the dosage based on symptoms from the previous administration. This substantially reduces the risk of side effects. In addition an IV of vitamin C (25 grams) immediately prior to the DMPS will reduce the risk of side effects. Never take any mercury chelator if you are constipated. DMPS can be administered in four ways:

1. *IV – Injecting DMPS into the blood stream.* Typically this is used to find out how much mercury your body is dumping. Research has indicated most of the chelation happens in the first six hours but through this method mercury can be eliminated for up to 24 hours. It is important to use this method at least every 4th time you get DMPS, and probably much more frequently. This provides the best chelation of mercury from your kidney. And the kidney stores a vast amount of mercury.

2. *IM – Injecting DMPS into a muscle.* This allows the DMPS to work longer with a range of 3 to 5 days. This is the preferred method for many

patients who want the maximum effect from DMPS; however it is also the riskiest and has the potential for the most side effects. Do not use DMPS IM until you have been able to tolerate DMPS IV at least five times without side effects, and have slowly built up to the maximum dosage. In IM and IV administration, DMPS should be given every 7-10 days for three cycles then eliminate it for three weeks before starting the cycle again.

3. *Oral – Swallowing a 250mg DMPS tablet.* This has value once you are well into the detoxification process. The tablet is only 40% absorbed thus the other 60% flows through the intestines and can pick up mercury in the digestive tract. For patients that have digestive problems associated with mercury this makes a great deal of sense as part of your protocol. Typically the oral method is given for 5-7 days with two weeks off before starting again. In concert with this protocol, eat lots of fiber and get a colonic on the last day of the protocol. This will maximize the elimination of mercury. If you are constipated be sure to take herbs that create elimination at least twice per day.

4. *Neural – Injecting DMPS with procaine into various parts of the body.* This can be used in conjunction with IV or IM. In other words, your doctor may take some of the 5cc's (if that's the dosage based on various test results, body weight etc) and use it for his neural procedure. Neural therapy is great if your thyroid is causing problems. Your doctor will inject directly into both sides of the thyroid. Typical points to hit are scars, sinus areas, tonsils, joints etc. Be sure your doctor is an expert in neural therapy. This can be a very uncomfortable 15 minutes even with the very best practitioners, let alone someone just learning. This will provide relief in a specific area and should be used periodically. This is a great way to restore normal thyroid function. Most traditional doctors believe, when a thyroid is not functioning properly the only path is synthetic thyroid extract. This is absolutely not true. A thyroid once unburdened from mercury can restore functionality without prescription drugs.

As mentioned, get a vitamin and mineral IV after any DMPS procedure. Your doctor is going to suggest when to do this and design a "recipe" of vitamins and minerals that are tailored to your symptoms. Obviously, all the vitamins and minerals are important after a DMPS treatment. However in order to eliminate mercury that was stirred up by the DMPS, you should include as much vitamin C as you and your doctor are comfortable with at that point in your detoxification process. Many studies suggest that you can take as much as 75 grams of vitamin C in an IV without concern (however it is unlikely your doctor will prescribe this amount). This quantity insures that you will chelate additional metals from your system. The only side effect of this much vitamin C is that you will be very thirsty for 24 hours or so after the IV. Just drinks lots of water. In addition a colonic should be included after any DMPS protocol.

Hyaluronic acid (HA) is a carbohydrate found in most organs and tissues. It has been discovered that HA is a potentialating agent and when given with DMPS increases mercury elimination by two to four times. It is non-toxic and thus risk free.

There are other chelating agents that can be used to eliminate mercury from your body. However, none of them seem to have the same effect that DMPS has shown. BAL is used in the United States for severe mercury detoxification. However BAL can have some very severe side effects. The primary side effects are hypertension, nausea, vomiting and headaches.

Penicillamine is a distant derivative of penicillin and can be used in mild cases of mercury poisoning, but it also has been associated with a few side effects. Also care must be taken with individuals who are allergic to penicillin. It is interesting that penicillamine is often a drug of choice for MS patients. It alleviates certain symptoms in MS patients. Interesting or therapeutic?

EDTA is a chelator that is often used in lead poisoning. Some doctors use it for all heavy metals. Recent research suggests EDTA can in fact actually "drive" mercury further into your tissues and increase the toxicity of mercury if you are acutely poisoned. Research by Boyd Haley at the University of Kentucky suggests EDTA creates an environment that inhibits the enzyme process. **NEVER use EDTA to chelate mercury**. It is a very good chelator of lead; however, DMSA is better and provides the benefit of also chelating mercury.

EDTA is delivered by IV and orally. There is very little value of ever using EDTA IV for heavy metal chelation. There is some literature that supports EDTA orally after mercury has been removed. The benefit of the oral dosage is that EDTA will attract lead, aluminum, cadmium, and tin and have very little impact on important minerals, such as zinc. Thus, other than normal supplementation, it is a painless methodology to eliminate certain metals if they still show up on your hair analysis after the mercury is gone. The only adjustment I would make is add some additional zinc if using the oral form of EDTA. Recently some companies have started marketing EDTA via suppositories. In theory this is an excellent way to get EDTA. Up to 750 ml of EDTA enters the blood stream via the colon wall. Eventually research might support this as the best option for getting the benefits of EDTA

DMSA is a good mercury chelator, but it purportedly crosses the blood brain barrier. There is a great amount of debate on this issue and whether DMSA actually crosses the blood brain barrier. It is best to assume it does. This means, in theory that DMSA could actually move mercury from part of your body and dump it into your brain. Obviously this is a concern and DMSA should not be used until DMPS has eliminated most of the mercury from your body. Some doctors like to use DMSA "to mop up" residual mercury that DMPS may have missed or to address neurological symptoms. DMSA should be used part of your detoxification protocol as soon as mercury levels are reduced. Often doctors will alternate between DMPS and DMSA. There are numerous dosage protocols for DMSA but it seems most agree that 750 mg three times per day for 5 days then off for 14 days provides benefits. There have been very few reported cases of side effects but caution is appropriate with DMSA also. Start with lower dosages and work to the maximum. However, there can be just as many problems if the dosage is to low thus mobilizing metals but not eliminating them. Most, but not all practitioners do not feel it is necessary to get a vitamin and mineral IV after DMSA. But if you feel tired after a round of DMSA, get the IV, it can not hurt, otherwise just add additional minerals for a few days. Be sure to drink lots of water.

DMSA is great at eliminating aluminum, copper and lead. It is not unusual for patients to aggressively eliminate mercury but still have problem metals remain. If your hair analysis shows low mercury levels, but remaining metals such as those mentioned, they can be eliminated with DMSA and with very few side effects. Take the above dosage recommendation until other metals have been eliminated. Alternating between oral EDTA (once **all** the mercury has been eliminated) and DMSA would provide a valuable protocol in order to remove excess copper, lead, aluminum and lead.

DMPS and DMSA target particular organs. DMPS targets the kidneys, blood, and to a lesser extent the liver. DMSA attracts mercury in the liver, brain, spleen, intestines and muscles.

Alpha lipoic acid (ALA) is available in any health food store and is an excellent chelator when combined with DMPS or DMSA. Do not use it with either of the above chelators initially. Using it concert with one of the above chelators early might cause side effects. However after three to six months of DMPS or DMSA and in conjunction with a reduction in symptoms ALA will help the clean up process. ALA crosses the blood brain barrier, and in conjunction with DMSA is excellent at addressing neurological issues. But first decrease the mercury burden with DMPS. Use ALA in conjunction with the chelator (DMPS, and DMSA) and during "off times" stop the ALA as well. The dosage is variable, depending on the individual, but 100-500 mgs 3 times per day is a starting point. Evaluate your sense of wellness and increase or decrease the dosage based on how you feel.

VITAMINS AND MINERALS TO ASSIST IN DETOXIFICATION

You must supplement a number of vitamins and minerals daily. An important point to remember is that while you are on DMPS do not take zinc or chromium. But take all other vitamins. As a general guideline you should never take copper as part of your multi-vitamin. Due to the composition of your mercury amalgam you are probably copper toxic as well as mercury toxic. Your body does not need extra copper in any form. DMPS will bind to the excess copper and remove it from your system. DMPS has a strong affinity for both zinc and chromium and if you are taking them in concert with taking DMPS the DMPS might bind to them and not mercury. Thus if you get DMPS via IV do not take these minerals for 1 day, if you get DMPS IM then hold off on these minerals for 3 days, and orally wait two days after the completion of your cycle. It is not necessary to eliminate any minerals if you are using DMSA.

Before discussing vitamins, a brief discussion of heavy metals is appropriate. Mercury, nickel, lead and aluminum, arsenic, and cadmium all have a density of at least five times water. Heavy metals cannot be metabolized by the body, and they have no function. They should not be part of any diet. Yet some companies that sell vitamins include them in their formula. A well-known large manufacturer of vitamins has a multi vitamin that contains both nickel and tin. Nickel is a known carcinogen.

If a marketer of vitamins puts heavy metals in its product it is a product you should avoid. As a consumer you better read labels carefully. If you take a bad product in an effort to get well it will be like jumping from the fire to the frying pan.

Specifically what supplements do you need to take and in what quantities do you need to take them?

A Multi-vitamin needs to be is free of all corn, yeast, soy and wheat is the most important priority. In 2002 the AMA advised everyone to take a multi vitamin. However even if your vitamin contains all the various minerals and meets recommended daily allowances it won't be enough. I have no idea how anyone arrives at RDA's but the traditional RDA's do not meet your nutritional needs. You need to augment your multi-vitamin. In addition the multi-vitamin should not contain copper or iron.

Iron is complex and often times overlooked by doctors. Suffice to say very few people are deficient in iron. However many absorb too much iron and create an overloaded condition. Everyone should have a complete iron blood test before beginning any detoxification program. Excess iron can mimic mercury toxicity. This excess is deposited in the liver, pancreas, adrenals, heart, skeletal muscle, brain and creates many symptoms that are identical to the problems created by mercury. There is only way a person can become iron toxic; from increased intestinal absorption of iron. This is typically due to hemochromatosis, a genetic disorder affecting mainly males over 40 years of age with Irish, German or English heritage.

Removing the excess iron should be done as soon as possible. EDTA is an excellent chelator of iron and this can be administered in a variety of ways. The other option is phlebotomy. Drawing blood and thus releasing red blood cells that contain iron produces the same results as chelating the metal. Excess storage of iron in organs can result in irreversible damage. Thus it is important to quickly and effectively reduce iron overload.

Vitamin C is a powerful antioxidant, and it is valuable as you fight the effects of mercury. It is also a mild chelating agent and will help flush mercury, lead and copper from your body. Linus Pauling recommended huge quantities of vitamin C. And these recommendations assumed a reasonably healthy individual. If this is the case can you imagine how much you need if you are toxic? An illustration of this fact is that overloading with vitamin C orally causes diarrhea. However in order to induce diarrhea in toxic individuals often times it takes huge amounts of vitamin C, up to 70 grams. In healthy individuals it takes far less vitamin C. I know some doctors who actually use this fact as a test to determine if patients are toxic. If you want to try it; take 4 grams of buffered vitamin C powder mixed in water every 15-20 minutes. Do this until you get active diarrhea. You should achieve your goal of diarrhea after 20-30 grams of vitamin C. If it takes more than 30 grams of vitamin C then you can bet that you are toxic. There is a direct relationship between how much vitamin C is required and how toxic you are, and I think this relationship extends to how long it should take to get well. Do not use the vitamin C flush without discussing it with your doctor. If you are toxic, once active diarrhea starts it can continue for 12-24 hours. So be careful and be sure your doctor is available on the day you decide to try this protocol.

On a daily basis take at least 6-15 grams of vitamin C spread throughout the day. You can increase vitamin C to bowel tolerance without harm. However if you can spread the dosages such that you can take vitamin C every 2-3 hours taking the upper limit of the range will help you detoxify faster. One side effect of vitamin C is that it might magnify a condition called acidosis. Simply put this means the pH of your tissue becomes acidic. This can happen to mercury toxic people and if it does, you will need to reduce the amount of vitamin C you are taking or buy a pH neutral vitamin C.

Vitamin C enters every cell and is part of a process that creates glutathione. This is an amino acid that is critical in the detoxification process. It is also important for appropriate adrenal function.

Vitamin E is another antioxidant that should be taken during your detoxification. Typically 400-800 I.U. will suffice. Vitamin E does a couple of things. It protects vitamin A and in conjunction with glutathione, selenium and vitamin C, will protect your system from some of the toxic effects of mercury.

Selenium is an important trace mineral to add. 100-200 mcg per day will suffice. Many studies have demonstrated that selenium works synergistically with vitamin E to reduce the toxic effects of mercury. One of the reasons fish do not die from mercury poisoning is that they have huge amounts of selenium. It appears selenium binds to mercury making it inert. That's the good news; the bad news is that when bound the mercury may not readily exit the body. Selenium also increases the ratio of HDL to LDL. More is not better when taking selenium. Do not exceed 200 mcgs per day. Selenium can be toxic at high levels.

Zinc is a critical mineral that needs to be part of your supplementation program. Mercury will always reduce your zinc content. And the opposite is also true. As you increase your cellular level of zinc you will be able to more efficiently eliminate all heavy metals. Zinc is a precursor to many detoxification enzymes. Metallothioneins are intracellular proteins that provide a storage facility for zinc and also attract metals. Metallothioneins are comprised of sulfur based amino acids (primarily cysteine). Whenever mercury is attached to this SH molecule, since it has a higher affinity for mercury than zinc, zinc will be released and mercury will bind to the metallothioneins. The protective function of these small proteins is critical as we attempt to disarm the toxic effects of mercury.

If your hair analysis suggests low zinc levels this can be confirmed by testing for zinc in a blood plasma test. If both suggest low zinc then supplementation is critical. Taking a total of 30 mg of zinc per day is typically recommended. However if your hair analysis illustrates a very poor zinc level you can take up to 150 mgs without concern. The additional 130 mgs can make a huge difference in how you feel. Dosages up to 200 mgs per day, for short periods of time, are sometimes used in severely toxic patients. There are no known toxic effects at these levels if used for a short period of time. This additional zinc also helps chelate lead and copper. Zinc is an excellent chelator of lead and probably every mercury toxic individual is also lead toxic. Typically as zinc increases lead and copper will decrease.

After DMPS therapy, add extra zinc for a few days to replace the zinc that was lost during DMPS chelation. Zinc is lost since DMPS has an affinity for zinc and will not only bind to mercury but also zinc.

An interesting correlation between zinc and copper has been discovered. If you are zinc deficient you are probably also copper toxic. As long as this condition exists take extra zinc and be sure none of your supplements contain copper. The only potential side effect of extra zinc for an extended period of time is that cholesterol levels will probably increase, including LDL, while HDL decreases. Be sure to have periodic cholesterol checks if you are trying to raise zinc levels. Later in the book the value of a liver cleanse will be discussed and one of the benefits is that cleaning out stones will reduce cholesterol. But raising zinc levels is absolutely necessary in order to restore health.

If, after a few months taking a variety of doses of zinc, and zinc levels have not increased the problem is absorption. A few areas that should be considered:

1. A normal functioning pancreas and liver are necessary for zinc absorption.
2. Iron as well as copper will compete with zinc.
3. Adequate levels of trytophan (an amino acid) are necessary for absorption.
4. Elevated levels of chromium and manganese lowers zinc levels.
5. B12 is low.
6. HCL levels are low.

Try taking a pancreatic enzyme and a pancreatic glandular product and if your amino acid profile shows decreased trytophan add it to your list of products to take. Also, it may be necessary to abandon a multi-vitamin since they all include manganese and chromium. If both are elevated in your hair analysis and zinc is not increasing it will be necessary to eliminate manganese and chromium. This is a real challenge that is difficult for patients. Without a multi-vitamin it is necessary to supplement vitamins and minerals separately. If copper is high, that will inhibit zinc absorption, DMSA will chelate copper as will the amino acid arginine, and histidene. Lowering copper is necessary in order to increase zinc levels.

B12 is critical for absorption of all vitamins and minerals. And it is used in huge amounts during detoxification. It is involved in all types of methylation reactions. If you discover that nothing seems to be improving on subsequent hair tests then it is possible that B12 is the culprit. Intestinal dysbiosis (yeast and anaerobic bacteria in unbalanced amounts in your intestinal track) and the absence of intrinsic factor will cause B12 deficiencies. Low thyroid and poor adrenal function also reduces B12 absorption. These symptoms are all common in mercury toxic individuals and require B12 supplementation. Only small amounts of B12 are necessary but it is possible that levels have been depleted during any period of prolonged illness. In healthy individuals the liver can store up to 5 years of required B12. B12 is required for proper digestion, the synthesis of proteins (including methionine), it protects the fatty sheaths that cover nerve endings, it is integral in the immune systems ability to combat viruses and bacteria, it processes fatty acids, it is needed in phase 1 detoxification, and in the overall detoxification of toxins, and it activates important enzymes.

Symptoms of B12 deficiency, regardless of cause (heavy metals, bacteria, the absence of intrinsic value, viruses, leaky gut, anticoagulant drugs such as heparin, etc) will create the following symptoms; fatigue, digestive disorders, enlargement of the liver, nervousness, burning sensations often in the feet, and general neurological issues.

The solution is to get B12 shots, or take B12 sublingually. The oral form is not well absorbed. The shots are best. Dosage is individual specific. But up to 60 mgs per day have been given without significant adverse impact. Very few if any will ever need a dosage even close to that amount. But low B12 levels are often missed by practitioners in the detoxification process of mercury. The caution is to be sure that B12 does not increase cobalt levels. And if taking B12 in any fashion be sure to take folic acid. B12 and folic acid are synergistic and need to be taken together. Dosages should be directed by a doctor. The one caveat regarding B12 is histamine levels should be checked prior to any B12 therapy. If histamine levels are low B12 will make you feel like you have found the fountain of youth. If histamine levels are high B12 will have the exact opposite effect. If addition, histamine levels will effect all vitamins, minerals and herbs that effect methylation. This will be discussed in the section on amino acids and particularly its effect on methionine.

Finally, as noted earlier, make sure you have adequate HCL levels. It is impossible to absorb zinc without stomach acid. If you supplement zinc and HCL is absent, then zinc will simply be eliminated and copper levels will increase. Always take zinc (plus all other vitamins and minerals) with your primary meals. The goal is to recognize zinc increasing gradually. It may take years to finally achieve adequate levels, but progress should be seen in a few months.

B Complex provides numerous benefits, including energy, cellular repair, hormone production and adrenal function. Your multi vitamin probably does not provide enough B complex. Add a 50mg tablet twice per day. To maximize the benefit of B vitamins inject inter-muscularly a B vitamin complex once per week, up to 1cc. Most doctors will provide you a vile so that you can administer the injection yourself a couple of times per week.

B1 aids digestion and carbohydrate metabolism as well as brain function. Often mercury toxic individuals will have an enlarged liver...this is due to a deficiency in B1. B2 plays a major role in the formation of red blood cells and helps oxygenate tissues, a typical deficiency will demonstrate itself in cracks in the lips. B3 is a critical brain vitamin; it enhances memory. It plays a key role in the production of HCL and digestion. B5 aids in adrenal function and cholesterol production. B6 is probably the most important B vitamin. It assists brain function, helps regulate blood sugar issues, mediates heart disease, and is critical for a healthy nervous system. B12 and folic acid are discussed in a previous section. They deserve their own section based on importance. **B VITAMINS ARE VERY IMPORTANT. DON'T IGNORE THEM.**

Beta-carotene is an efficient anti-oxidant that everyone should be taking as part of a daily supplement. It protects against cancer and heart disease. A supplement with 25,000 I.U. will suffice.

Probiotics restore the good gut bugs your system needs. Many people theorize that good health starts in your gut. Thus it's fair to say that bad health may start in your gut.

Now, here are a few facts about the digestive system that are helpful. 70% of the immune function is located in the intestinal tract, and the digestive organs, the small intestine is about 23 feet in length. The inner surface of the small intestine is comprised of villi, which provides for the absorption of vitamins and minerals, the large intestine is about 5 feet in length. Your intestinal lining will regenerate every 3-5 days. Approximately 100,000,000,000 bacteria inhabit the intestinal tract.

Most mercury toxic people have gut problems of some type. The reason is that mercury has changed the flora of your digestive system and bad gut bugs are thriving and the good guys are losing the battle. Mercury kills friendly bacteria and causes some bacteria to mutate. In order to reinforce your good gut bugs take large amounts of a probiotic that includes both acidophilus and bifidus. Triple or even quadruple the recommended dosage. One study states the total probiotic taken should equal 10 billion organisms (and this might be low). The probiotic should require refrigeration as well as be enterically coated so it passes thru stomach acid and bile without harm. The more strains the probiotic has, the better. Continue increasing the dosage until you have normal digestion. In my case I used 16 times the recommended dosage until I was able to balance the bacteria in my gut. Also be sure to find a probiotic that is dairy-free. If you are taking any type of antibiotic the greater the amount of probiotic you take the better. Antibiotics play havoc with not only the bacteria they are trying to kill, but also the bacteria in your intestinal tract. It is absolutely mandatory to constantly replace bacteria that might have been killed by any antibiotic.

Saccro boulardi is beneficial yeast that should be taken with your probiotic. It will help balance gut flora and have a negative effect on the harmful bacteria in the gut. Beta Glutan is a relative of to Saccro B and studies suggests it stimulates the immune system.

Unbalanced or unhealthy bacteria in the intestinal tract is the cause of disease. Dysbiosis is the label given to an unhealthy balance of bacteria. This leads to leaky gut syndrome, which is an inflammation of the intestinal tract and a breakdown in the integrity of the intestinal wall. In healthy individuals tiny openings in the intestinal tract allows vitamins and minerals to enter the blood stream. As inflammation happens, these openings allow foreign material (large proteins) to enter the bloodstream. This creates an immune response as well as liver stress. It leads to perceived food allergies and other symptoms based on foreign material entering the blood stream. Insuring a healthy digestive system is critical for recovery. Hippocrates stated, "Man is not nourished by what he swallows but by what he digests and uses." This statement is 21st century wisdom as it applies to detoxification. Simply stated; take huge amounts of probiotics.

Grapefruit seed extract. In conjunction with acidophilus, grapefruit seed extract helps repair your gastric system. This simple product combats unhealthy gastric flora better than anything you can purchase. It will destroy excess yeast without serious die off problems. Depending on the severity of your symptoms, take 2-4 capsules per day.

Magnesium. All mercury toxic people are magnesium deficient. Not some, but all, are deficient. I suggest that you test this theory by getting magnesium push (IV) and see how you feel afterwards. Most people feel markedly better for a short time. This push can be done in concert with a vitamin IV after a DMPS or DMSA protocol. Typically it is done combining magnesium and procaine. Up to 400mg of magnesium can be used without concern. If this helps, generally or specifically, get a magnesium push periodically. It will help your overall sense of well being and specifically helps eliminate joint pain. Then as part of your daily supplements take a well absorbed magnesium. Magnesium glycinate is an excellent choice. Recommended dosages are 400-600 mgs per day. Assuming bowel tolerance, you can triple this dosage without concern. And often times the increased dosage will have a profound and positive effect on how you feel. If one of your symptoms is anxiety, this is often times correlated with a magnesium deficiency. Try taking additional magnesium and see if the anxiety improves. Other symptoms of magnesium deficiency are fatigue, muscle aches, high blood pressure, sugar cravings and insomnia. Some believe a craving for chocolate is actually just the need for magnesium. Chocolate is high in magnesium.

Magnesium is involved in over 300 enzymatic reactions. It is critical in the protein production process, is needed for GSH synthesis which is used in phase 2 detoxification, is involved in the production of hormones, effects the production of ATP, and is needed in the production of HCL along with potassium. Deficiencies will cause TSC to increase along with elevated levels of LDL and reduced levels of HDL.

Many symptoms improve once optimum levels of magnesium are achieved. However be aware it might take years to fully correct a magnesium deficiency. And do not take magnesium at the same time as calcium or calcium rich foods.

Calcium. Calcium is synergistic with magnesium. In all probability you are getting plenty of calcium in your multi and the vegetables you eat. Do not supplement additional calcium.

Vitamin A. Taking between 25000-50000 IU per day for the first month or so of detoxification is appropriate. Then decrease to 15000 to 25000 IU per day until your symptoms are gone. Vitamin A protects membranes from toxins and this is important in your detoxification process. But be careful, Vitamin A is toxic in high doses. If you are pregnant consult with a physician before taking increased amounts of Vitamin A.

Manganese. If your hair analysis shows decreased manganese, take an additional dose of manganese. This is trace mineral that competes with mercury and often time's mercury toxic individuals are deficient in manganese. Manganese and zinc are antagonistic minerals. If one is high the other is low. For example, if zinc is low manganese will be elevated. If this occurs avoid manganese in all forms. Otherwise it will be very difficult to normalize zinc.

Silymarin. Often called milk thistle this will help detoxify the liver. It is a very powerful herb that is a great antioxidant. It prevents liver cell damage and aids in regenerating liver cell damage. Three 100mg tablets per day should be enough.

Garlic and Alfalfa. These are all excellent products that will assist your body in recovering from the effects of mercury poisoning. Mercury will bind to the amino acids in these products and be eliminated from your body. Garlic is high in sulfur and is a very important herb to take while detoxifying. As opposed to buying garlic tablets, buy organic garlic and eat 1-2 cloves per day. This is more effective, and far less expensive than any garlic pill. Alfalfa is very alkaline and should be used. Chorella and various forms of algae and spirulina are sometimes used to chelate mercury. The problem with each of them is that they are grown in the sea and are contaminated with mercury. If you decide to take chorella be sure the manufacturer can produce information showing that the product is free from any toxins, including mercury. If the assay is not available or shows any level of mercury avoid the product.

Broad spectrum parasite cleanse. This combination of herbs helps rid your system of parasites. It's a good bet that a variety of parasites have taken up residence in your body. As you release mercury from your system this cleanse will help release parasites, and their toxins such that proper intestinal health can be reestablished. A good cleanse takes 90 days.

Essential fatty acids. EFA's are critical for cell membrane structure, and they transform into local hormones. EFA imbalances often create a variety of inflammatory conditions. The American diet consists almost solely of omega 6 oils. The ideal ratio of omega 6 to omega 3 is about 4:1, estimates today suggest the actual ratio is 20:1. Most saturated fats (omega 6) raise cholesterol levels while omega 3 increases cell permeability, and provides benefits to the muscular skeletal system, heart and the entire endocrine system.

87

The best source of omega 3 EFA is fish oil. Eating fish to get this benefit is a terrible option since all fish are contaminated with mercury. But most fish oil does not contain mercury. MegaOmega, Biotics and Metagenics produce fish oil that has been assayed and is mercury free, or very low in mercury. These are good products produced by good companies. However the fish oil marketed by Dr. Sears claims to have less PCB's and mercury than any other product. Fish oil is a great source of omega 3, DHA and EPA. Flaxseed is another terrific source but enzymes must convert the EFA to DHA and EPA. This process is often compromised by mercury. Include plenty of fish oil every day. One study demonstrated high doses of omega 3 reduce depression in people who demonstrated this symptom. Other studies show omega 3 reduces heart disease. This could be due to the fact that omega 3 lowers LDL and raises HDL. Other food sources of omega 3 are all nuts and seeds.

Digestive enzymes. Again you should use enzymes if your digestive system is compromised. This protocol can have a very positive effect very quickly. If mercury has invaded your digestive tract, and I'll bet it has, then using digestive enzymes is a requirement. One of the problems in your intestinal tract is that magnesium is required to complete the enzyme cycle. If mercury has replaced magnesium then it's impossible to get the proper enzyme balance. Until you eliminate mercury you will need to supplement with enzymes. Take a good digestive enzyme with all meals, and snacks. A good digestive enzyme includes the following; protease, amylase, lipase, cellulose, sucrase, lactase and maltase.

When enzymes are at optimal levels, proper digestion and nutrient absorption takes place. In addition, detoxification is also more efficient. Processed foods and cooking eliminate enzymes. Raw fruit and vegetables provide a powerful supply of enzymes. Health cannot be restored and detoxification cannot take place without enzymes. Supplement at every meal.

In addition to enzymes add a daily fiber product. Do not take any fiber supplement if you are constipated. Add herbal products to remedy the constipation problem then add a fiber supplement. Drink 16-24 oz. of water for every glass of fiber product that you take. Your fiber supplement, in addition to the vegetables and fruits you are eating will decrease transit time in your intestinal track and insure that any mobilized mercury is not reabsorbed in your gut. Decreasing transit time during detoxification is a primary objective. You should be targeting 30-50 grams of fiber per day. It is impossible to reach this target without a fiber supplement.

Coenzyme Q10. This is neither a vitamin nor mineral, but there is some compelling research that suggests everyone should be taking 60 mgs per day. If you have heart disease 200 mgs per day is recommended. CoQ10 is a fat-soluble nutrient found in every cell of the body. CoQ10 stimulates the immune system and is very helpful for people who have multiple chemical sensitivity and all types of allergies. It also oxygenates cells.

Aloe Vera. This is a powerful detoxifier and will stimulate your immune system. Additionally, studies have demonstrated a positive correlation between aloe vera and T lymphocytes. The aloe vera that is available in stores will not be effective; you need a far greater concentration. T-Up produces an aloe vera that is excellent. It tastes horrible but is concentrated and very effective.

MSM. In addition to the above vitamins, minerals and herbs, consider supplementing with Methyl-sulfonyl-methane, commonly called MSM. MSM is a naturally occurring sulfur compound that is found in every tissue, cell and fluid in the human body. MSM creates flexible arteries, which allows oxygen to pass thru walls and nourish tissues.

Sulfur is just as critical to life as oxygen, magnesium or the B vitamins. It is very likely you are deficient in sulfur, since processing procedures, overcooking and mineral deficient soil all rob foods of sulfur. In addition, sulfur is secreted in huge amounts as part of the mercury detoxification process. MSM assists the digestive process, and is part of the process the liver uses to secrete bile. This is critical in the detoxification process.

Supplementing with MSM provides a foundation for better health and assists your body in detoxification. If your hair analysis shows decreased sulfur levels, MSM helps. Amino acids help, and those will be discussed in the next chapter. MSM is very inexpensive and adding 2-20 grams per day is a worthwhile option. If your hair analysis shows even a small deficiency in sulfur high dosages of MSM will be necessary. Start slowly and increase the dosage gradually. You need the sulfur and MSM is non toxic. Any excess will be flushed out in 12-24 hours.

MSM research has shown that many illnesses improve with supplementation of between 250-5000 mgs. The illnesses include

89

environmental allergies, food allergies, arthritis, constipation, conjunctivitis, and muscle pain. It is best to divide your daily dosage equally throughout the day. And it may take 12-24 months before you see results and changes in symptoms.

SOD. This is a powerful antioxidant and should be used to combat free radicals in any form. It is effective when viral or bacterial infection exists and for any form of inflammation. Most research suggests that granulated forms of SOD absorb more effectively than capsules or tablets.

Electrolyte drinks. This is not a reference to Gatorade, but to the opportunity to add electrolytes to water. Drinking water is the foundation all good health, and insuring that lost electrolytes are added back to the body is very important. There are many manufacturers that produce an electrolyte product that contains potassium, phosphorous, chloride, magnesium and sulfur that is simply added to a glass of water. This only increases the value of the glass of water that you are drinking. It is very useful if you are using any form of sweat therapy as part of your detoxification process. It is a very inexpensive way to insure that you are replacing electrolytes.

IAG. This a trade name for a product produced by Biotics. If a sophisticated blood chemistry is done and it included natural killer cell function, in all probability it will show a compromised immune system. In order to attain optimum health, it is important to have a healthy functioning immune system. It is necessary to enhance and improve the natural killer cells in your body. IAG is extracted from the western larch tree and is known as one of the herbs that can quickly and effectively improve immune function. Any herb that improves immune function should be part of the detoxification process. Not because the herb will help remove mercury but because as you improve your immune function you will naturally detoxify without the use of chemicals and other methodologies.

There are numerous manufacturers of vitamins and minerals. Most are not worth the money. Most products that are sold in grocery stores etc are not tested for bioavailability, toxic metals and contaminants. Basically you get what you pay for. From my experience the best professional products are: Thorne, Biotics, Standard Process, and Metagenics, and not necessarily in that order. Depending on symptoms and needs, it may be necessary to use all four. Be wary of doctors that only use a single source of vitamins. Call each manufacturer and get a catalog or ask your doctor for one. Vitamins and minerals will be an expensive proposition, make sure you are spending your money wisely. Make the choice of which vitamins, minerals, herbs etc you are going to take in conjunction with your doctor. For most clinics selling products is a profit center. The mark up is anywhere from 50-200%, thus if you can find a way to buy the products you need wholesale then do so. Determine the products you want to use and then shop for the best price. Be informed, be smart and spend your money wisely.

Remember the four critical thoughts:

.. DON'T BELIEVE TRADITIONAL MD'S REGARDING MERCURY. They are wrong.
.. DETOXIFYING FROM MERCURY IS A PROCESS, NOT AN EVENT. It takes time, in some cases, years.
.. LEARN EVERYTHING YOU CAN FROM THIS BOOK AND OTHER SOURCES OF INFORMATION. Become an expert.
.. DON'T GIVE UP. Stay with the process of detoxification. You will see improvement eventually.

CHAPTER 8

Buy The Truth And Do Not Sell It; Get Wisdom, Discipline And Understanding

AMINO ACIDS, THE MISSING SUPPLEMENT

Amino acids are the building blocks for proteins; they are essential for life. Amino acids are just as essential as oxygen, sulfur and hydrogen. There are 22 amino acids, but only eight are classified as essential since they can create the remaining amino acids through metabolic processes. Mercury can create a logjam in these enzymatic processes creating an amino acid imbalance, which makes metabolic transformation impossible. This typically occurs in the critical process of detoxification for many patients. The detoxification process is the role of the liver. Amino acids form over 1600 basic proteins which are used to create hormones, enzymes and antibodies.

The eight essential amino acids are isoleucine, leucine, lysine, methionine, phenylaline, threonine, trytophan, and valine. From these eight amino acids, the human body makes the other 15 amino acids. It is possible, if you read another book to classify some amino acids as semi-essential. Suffice to say the terminology is confusing. All 23 are essential to a healthy life. The body requires all 23 in order to survive. The eight mentioned must be obtained from a food source or a supplement since they cannot be made via a metabolic process, thus they are labeled essential. Amino acids are comprised of nitrogen, carbon, oxygen, hydrogen, and in some cases sulfur. Adequate levels of all 23 amino acids are necessary for the absorption and utilization of vitamins. Amino acids are the transport vehicles for vitamins and if there are deficiencies in the amino acids, then vitamins are not properly utilized.

In order to determine an amino acid profile it is best to order a comprehensive amino acid report. It is possible for a laboratory to obtain results from urine or plasma. The urine analysis is less expensive but far less accurate. Order the plasma test, it requires a 12 hour fast. In some cases your doctor might want both tests, since the combined results often provide better information than either test individually.

If your test shows a broad based deficiency, take an amino acid complex of all eight essential amino acids. Seven of the eight should be easily tolerated. If you have side effects from the comprehensive blend, eliminate methionine (which is the only sulfur based amino acid in the eight essential amino acids) then determine how you feel with just seven. In addition, supplement directly any non-essential amino acid that is more than 30% below the norm.

Earlier it was discussed that mercury has an affinity for sulfur. Methionine, along with cysteine, taurine, and glutathione are sulfur-based amino acids. Methionine is found in many foods and is critical in the detoxification process. However, due to the impact of mercury, methionine metabolism can be severely impaired. Supplementing with methionine, for some people who are acutely toxic can create problems.

Improper methionine metabolism creates homocysteine that is now considered a more serious precursor to heart disease than cholesterol or LDL. In theory, methionine converts to homocysteine and homocysteine then converts to other amino acids. When this pathway is blocked for whatever reasons the consequences can be serious. The most common symptom of methionine metabolism problems is fatigue. Other aberrant reactions are gastro issues, liver dysfunction, and muscle aches and pains. If your amino acid profile shows low amino acids, supplementation should create increased energy within a few days. If the opposite occurs, eliminate methionine. It is also possible that low histamine levels are the problem. This will be discussed in depth in Chapter 9 in the section on copper.

Methionine is a very important amino acid in the detoxification process and should be used as a supplement, if possible.

Methionine is a precursor to cysteine, glutathione, and taurine. It is absolutely critical to have adequate levels of the sulfur-based amino acids. They are crucial in detoxification, and if they are low, then detoxification is impossible. Taurine is easily tolerated in almost everyone regardless of the level of toxicity. Often times if methionine is a problem cysteine in any form will also be a problem. It has also been reported that oral DMSA can create many of the aberrant reactions that some of the sulfur based amino acids produce. If this is the case avoid all forms of cysteine as well as

DMSA. This means inspecting your vitamins to see if NAC is one of the components.

One of the ultimate goals is to create glutathione and, unfortunately, taking glutathione directly is a waste of money. Glutathione is made in the liver from other amino acids. Taken orally it is not well absorbed. However, taken in an IV it is easily absorbed.

Glutathione (GSH) is a powerful antioxidant and the most important amino acid in mercury detoxification. GSH is comprised of three amino acids: glycine, glutamic acid and cysteine. Complex metabolic processes produce the three. Thus it is complicated to create GSH. GSH is vital in liver detoxification, and declines naturally as we age, and it is also depleted as it detoxifies various toxins including mercury. In other words, in an ideal world we would like to have excess GSH, and in no circumstances do we want to have too little. But in most cases mercury toxic people are in that exact situation.

Since GSH is an SH molecule, mercury will inactivate the S (sulfur) portion of the molecule and thus GSH loses its detoxifying ability. This is a double-edge sword. The non-compromised GSH molecules detoxify mercury, while the compromised molecules lose their effectiveness due to mercury inactivating the sulfur portion of the molecule. For the above reasons, GSH must be replaced during detoxification. Protein and protein powders, brussel sprouts, garlic and red beets are all sources of GSH. Research indicates that it takes two GSH molecules to trap one mercury molecule for excretion. Once bound by GSH mercury is excreted via the feces. Thus it is impossible to supplement too much GSH. Creating GSH is critical, and without it detoxification is impossible. GSH is non toxic; the more the better.

The best source of GSH is whey protein. Immunocal is a trade name for an excellent whey protein. The web site is www.immunotec.com. It is important to take at least one packet of Immunocal every day. If the price of Immunocal is not within your budget, second choices would be other sources of non-denatured whey protein, NAC, (if it can be tolerated) glycine, taurine and glutamic acid, plus the food sources of GSH. Immunocal is listed in the PDR thus your physician can write a prescription for it. Foods that contain high levels of GSH are avocado, asparagus, paisley, lamb, and veal. GSH via IV is a great option but this is expensive. If possible, make Immunocal a very high priority on your list of supplements to take very day. GSH not only helps eliminate heavy metals but it also targets the liver and as the liver becomes healthier many symptoms including multiple chemical sensitivities will improve.

Another very important amino acid is glutamine. Glutamine is the most abundant amino acid and serves as transportation for nitrogen. Although not considered essential, i.e. available only from foods, it is essential during stages when usage exceeds availability. In other words you cannot make enough glutamine during periods of stress. It must be supplemented. Glutamine is critical for gastrointestinal tract integrity. Mercury disrupts the entire intestinal track creating dysbiosis and leading to leaky gut or intestinal permeability and glutamine is the best supplement for repair.

Large doses up to 20 grams are necessary if the amino acid results show low glutamine. Once the gut is repaired, absorption of vitamins and minerals is increased which provides additional benefits. One of the many frustrations patients experience is taking all the right vitamins and minerals but with seemingly no benefit. The reason is that absorption takes place in the gut. If intestinal permeability is an issue there is a great deal of wasting. Taking vitamins and minerals is critical to recovery but only if they are absorbed.

Since mercury has a negative effect on every organ including the heart, supplement carnitine if it shows a deficiency on the amino acid test.

The B vitamins, particularly B6 and B12, zinc, and magnesium are cofactors in amino acid metabolism. Since only B12 is difficult to absorb orally it is important to get enough from food. The other cofactors should be taken in oral form.

In addition to the essential amino acids, glutamine and GSH, take any amino acid that is deficient more than 30% from the norm, this is particularly important if tyrosine, taurine, tryptophan, and glycine are deficient. Glycine is an excellent chelator of aluminum and one of the three amino acids that comprise GSH. If your hair analysis demonstrates elevated aluminum it would be appropriate to supplement glycine. Tyrosine is an important amino acid that is primarily involved in the health of the thyroid gland. Carnitine is important since it strengthens the heart and regulates the delivery of trigicerides.

Without the benefit of amino acids, regaining health is impossible. This is often forgotten or ignored as part of most recovery processes, DO NOT IGNORE IT. Retake the amino acid profile every six months or so. This allows you to reestablish dosages. The only form of amino acid that should be supplemented is the L form. Amino acids are best absorbed when taken on an empty stomach. However with the amino acid take a small amount of natural sugar such as fruit juice and a small amount of protein. This enhances absorption.

THE DETOXIFICATION PATHWAYS

Once your mercury amalgams are removed, protocols are established to eliminate the toxins, and a supplement program is then established, it is important to understand how toxins actually exit our body. Mercury is eliminated four ways, skin (through sweating), kidneys (via urination), intestinal tract (through bowel movements), and liver (via bile). Use all four avenues to maximize getting the poison out.

SAUNAS

To the best of my knowledge, there are no reputable laboratories that economically measure sweat, but let us assume sweating is good and eliminates toxins. One of the problems for some people is that mercury creates intolerance to heat, and sweating is simply impossible. Typically these patients are the sickest and take the longest to recover. For those people, do not use a sauna until your body has detoxed enough such that you can sweat through exercise. For everyone else, the sauna is a good idea. Start slowly in both time and temperature and determine if the process promotes a sense of well-being or creates side effects of concern. If the sauna feels great, increase both the time spent in it and the temperature. Using it multiple times per day is the ultimate objective. Be sure to drink lots of liquids and take a cool shower after each session so you do not reabsorb the toxins that have been released. Be sure you replace the sodium and potassium that was lost as part of the sweating process. A good electrolyte drink, not to be confused with Gatorade, replaces all the minerals that were lost while in the sauna. The liquid, which is usually mixed with water, should contain sodium, potassium, phosphorous, chloride, magnesium and sulfur.

The best type of sauna to use, if you have options, is the infrared. It purportedly accesses deeper tissue for a more through detoxification. Use the sauna on a scheduled basis just like using a chelator. Sweating after DMPS or DMSA is a great idea.

In the mercury mines in Spain, every worker would leave the mines and go directly to the hospital and be placed under heat lamps in order to sweat and expel the mercury. Saunas are a 21st century solution to a 200-year-old problem.

In addition to the sauna, hot mineral baths are a great choice. Not every locale has access to natural mineral baths but they are hot and promote sweating. The baths contain phosphorous, calcium, sodium, potassium and zinc. Typically after the bath you are wrapped for 30 minutes to stimulate additional detoxification. Most places that have this wonderful natural product market it as relaxation. In reality, it is medicinal in that detoxification is a byproduct.

Finally, a simple and easy sweat is a hot bath with epsom salts. Make the water as hot as you can stand it, stay in for as long as you can, then if you get someone to wrap you stay wrapped and sweating for 20-30 minutes. If not, take a shower and appreciate that you eliminated toxins.

WATER AND AIR

Install a good water filtration system. Drink pure water, no fluoride, which is also a poison, or heavy metals that often times are in drinking water. Multi Pure makes a number of filters and some of them even guarantee to eliminate mercury from water. Regardless of what is installed, send a sample after installation to a water testing company and compare the results with the manufacturer claims. Once you have clean water drink it, 5-10 glasses a day. This is the best way to flush toxins from the kidney. Water keeps cells hydrated, which stimulates the elimination of waste products and toxins.

It is difficult to purify the air, but you should try. Use air cleaners in your furnace, room cleaners in rooms that you frequent, and an ozonator near an intake vent in your house. This will send ozone through out the house. Be sure windows are open when using the ozonator. Ozone is a powerful antibacterial. Also avoid petrochemicals as much as possible. Avoid natural gas heat, gasoline fumes, propane, and dry cleaning. Replace carpeting with hardwood floors. This reduces the workload of the liver.

Do not use pesticides on your lawn or plants and sleep with the window open in your room.

COLONICS ARE A VERY USEFUL PROTOCOL

Most tests today measure mercury elimination via the kidneys. However, most research that exists today suggests that the more mercury is eliminated through the intestines. The problem is that very few laboratories measure mercury output via the intestines. Mercury is stored in the intestines, and it is also eliminated through the colon. Additionally, it is fair to state that a healthy colon is critical in order to insure overall health. A healthy colon is essential for the absorption of vital nutrients and the elimination of body waste and toxins. A diseased or unhealthy colon guarantees illness. Colon cancer is the #2 cancer killer in the United States. It makes sense to keep it clean.

When colon function is sluggish, toxins are forced into the blood stream and circulate to every organ in the body. This compromises the immune system, and creates health problems and degenerative disease. Some health care professionals believe that the sickest people are people with inefficient elimination. These same practitioners list a lengthy list of symptoms associated with poor bowel movement that amazingly similar to the symptoms that present themselves in mercury toxic individuals.

Colonics use water for cleaning and rejuvenating every cell in the body. By removing fecal matter from the colon walls, bacteria and toxin levels are reduced. When toxin levels are reduced in the colon, the vascular and lymphatic system releases additional waste into the colon for further cleansing. This ongoing process helps detoxify your total body. Some German research suggests that highly toxic people need 50-300 colonics before full health can be restored. And this estimate might be low in very toxic individuals. Colonics help retrain the colon. As your colon regains health, your symptoms improve, bowel movements become more frequent, and oxygen levels rise.

A certified hydro-therapist who understands heavy metal toxicity is the preferred practitioner to use when doing colonics. Try and find someone with at least 3 years experience in heavy metal detoxification. The facility should be using FDA approved equipment. Also use a facility that uses gravity equipment. In addition, the herbs mentioned previously for parasites should be part of this protocol. If ozone is legal in your area and the colon hydro-therapist uses it, absolutely make it part of your protocol. Ozone contains three molecules of oxygen. It is therefore more reactive than oxygen and as one molecule breaks away the normal oxygen molecule remains. Ozone combats viruses, bacteria, breaks down chemicals and increases oxygenation in tissues and cells.

In order to maximize the benefits of DMPS or DMSA, colonics should be performed after each DMPS or DMSA treatment. If the DMPS treatment is via IV you should have a colonic 2-4 hours after the IV, IM every day for three days if possible, and oral DMPS or DMSA every day for the length of the protocol if possible. As part of your colonic, use a coffee implant and try to hold it for 15-20 minutes. Coffee stimulates bile elimination and this causes additional toxins to be released. After a colonic, take a comprehensive probiotic. Most practitioners will provide this to you before you leave their clinic, but it may not be enough. That night take additional probiotics.

The cost of a colonic depends on geography and the type of equipment that is used. If the cost and the projected cost of repeated colonics are prohibitive, substitute a coffee enema. This does not replicate the overall benefit of a colonic but an enema provides some benefit. An enema is a poor man's colonic. It stimulates the liver to release bile and therefore toxins. Be sure to fill the enema bag 5-7 times to receive the maximum benefit.

Often constipation is a problem. Colonics will help remedy this problem. In addition, Metagenics makes a number of powders that can be used during the detoxification process. UltraClear Sustain will help eliminate constipation. It is a great product for patients who suffer from constipation or irregular bowel movements.

THE LIVER – THE ULTIMATE FILTER

The liver is located just beneath the ribs on the right side, it weighs about 5 pounds and is the largest organ in your body. It is similar in size to a football, 8 inches long and 4 inches wide. The liver has over 500 functions but the most important to a reader of this book is detoxification. Other functions are blood sugar regulation, bile production, cholesterol production (which starts hormone production), carbohydrate conversion, breaking proteins into useable energy forms, stores Vitamin D, Vitamin A and B12 for future use, filters blood, removes toxins, bacteria, viruses and yeast, and producing enzymes. It is clear the liver is a very important organ, and it is important to support the liver in order to insure optimum efficiency and thus insure your optimum health.

The liver can remove mercury, and other heavy metals from the bloodstream, and excrete it through the bile it creates. The problem occurs when various chemicals, toxins, and heavy metals overload the liver's ability to detoxify the various poisons. When this happens, the body's filter is compromised and toxins, including mercury, are not released from the liver and this congestion backs up and affects every organ in the body.

The liver's detoxification process is labeled phase one and phase two. These are not necessarily unique separate phases, but have a number of common pathways. It is critical to have phase one and phase two "behaving" appropriately. The best description of phase one is that the liver prepares the toxin for elimination. It converts very toxic substances into a water soluble form that is less toxic for easier elimination. Phase two eliminates the toxin. For example, phase one is similar to dumping leftover food into the sink, cutting it into small pieces and mixing it with water. Phase two would be turning on the disposal.

Phase one is accomplished through a group of enzymes labeled P450 and phase two is accomplished by numerous mechanisms. Reduced P450 enzymes are associated with a low protein diet, low HCL, and reduced absorption of vitamins and minerals, such as zinc, magnesium, B6 and B12. Phase one produces free radicals and it is necessary to insure that adequate antioxidants are available or else these free radicals damage liver cells. The great news is that the liver can regenerate itself and any damage that has been caused to the liver will remedy itself in time. The damage is only temporary.

Phase two is a complex and integrated process that involves all the sulfur-based amino acids. It is necessary to have adequate supplies of all of them. The sulfur-based amino acids render the toxins harmless and release them via the bile produced by the liver. Great Smokies Laboratory, in its liver detoxification profile, measures four mechanisms or pathways in phase two; glutathione conjugation, glycine conjugation, sulfation, and glucuronidation. It is important that each is working optimally. Typically the sulfation pathway will be compromised when a person is mercury toxic.

When any portion of phase one or phase two is out of balance it will cause symptoms and free radical production. Each phase and pathway has complex and specific responsibilities. They all lead up to the final objective in Phase two. Prepare toxins for elimination by processing them into water-soluble metabolites.

Once phase one and phase two are operating efficiently the detoxification process will proceed much more quickly. Toxins can be rendered harmless and eliminated via bile assuming proper nutrients are available including the sulfur-based amino acids, particularly glutathione.

Mercury toxic individuals can exhibit any combination of liver functions. Every 9-12 months during detoxification individuals should have the liver test offered by Great Smokies Laboratory.

In addition to supporting the liver with phase one and phase two nutrients it is beneficial to do a liver cleanse. This simple task can unblock physical pathways and provide the liver an opportunity to continue its task of detoxifying a variety of toxins including mercury. A few indicators that suggest a sluggish liver are chemical sensitivities, fatigue, high cholesterol, fibromyalgia, blood sugar imbalances, digestive problems and neurological issues such as depression, memory problems, and irritability. A very predictable physical symptom of a sluggish liver is hemorrhoids. Also hemorrhoids often indicate a clotting problem and this often indicates an infection of some type. If you have hemorrhoids a liver cleanse should be a priority once you have the hemorrhoids removed. There are very simple procedures available that preclude hemorrhoid surgery that involve laser and electrical stimulation that "zap" the inflammation.

The purpose of a liver cleanse is to create free flowing bile and eliminate debris from the gallbladder. It is a very simple procedure that was once used at the Lahey Clinic in Boston. The objective is to get the gallbladder to release accumulated matter composed of stagnant bile, cholesterol, and toxins. For the first six days eat your normal diet and some type of natural acid is taken that softens hardened material in the gallbladder and liver. Often phosphoric acid is used.

On day six large amounts of magnesium are taken, which allows for the relaxation of the bile duct, thereby allowing stones to pass comfortably. In order to stimulate the release of the stones and sludge the evening of day six a natural oil is taken at bedtime usually olive oil, in a rather large quantity with grapefruit juice. Immediately after drinking the oil go to bed and lie on your right side and try to sleep. There will be a great deal of gurgling. Usually by 4-5 a.m. you will begin releasing the stones. The stones will be green, brown or black, and range in size from 1/16th of inch all the way to ¾ of an inch. The stones are being expelled from the gallbladder through the bile duct, into the colon and out of the body. During the process of elimination there may be periods of nausea but it will pass. This is simply the result of the contraction of the gallbladder and the release of toxins. The stones may be soft or hard and you may release hundreds of them on the morning of day 7. Most cleanses recommend a coffee enema on the morning of release but a colonic is much better. In addition to a normal colonic, stimulate additional release by rectally holding a quart of organic coffee for 15-20 minutes. When you release the coffee additional stones are released.

If you release hundreds of stones, do another cleanse in 2-3 weeks. Continue doing this cleanse until very few stones are being released. Then regardless of how well you feel, make a liver/gallbladder cleanse a regular part of your protocol. Most practitioners believe it should be done every six months. The result of the cleanse will be a sense of well-being. The day of the release you may be tired and if so try and get some sleep. But overall, you should experience a release from many symptoms and have improved energy. In order to find a cleanse that will work for you most facilities that provide colonics have a protocol and the necessary ingredients to accomplish your objective. In addition, naturopathic physicians and alternative medical doctors have some favorite protocols. Most are very similar but vary in some ways. Many use epsom salts as the magnesium on day 6 but this has been found to be toxic to the intestinal tract and magnesium citrate is now preferred.

A more benign cleanse that can be used combines 8 oz. of purified water, 8 oz. of juiced organic citrus, either orange or grapefruit, the juice of one lemon, and daily increase of olive oil, ginger, and garlic. On the morning of day one, take one tablespoon of olive oil, one garlic capsule, or one clove, and one ginger cap. Each successive morning for a total of five days, increase the olive oil by one tablespoon, and the garlic, or ginger by one capsule. On the afternoon of the fifth day have a colonic; small stones may be released. This liver cleanse will not produce the volume of stones when larger amounts of olive oil is used but it can be done more frequently, and is beneficial in purifying the liver and gallbladder.

If stones are being released you are probably magnesium deficient. Take 400-600 mgs of magnesium every day. In addition if the detoxification profile suggests liver pathway problems it is likely that adrenal function needs to be addressed. Finally the following amino acids are critical to a healthy liver; methionine, alanine, threonine, and arginine.

Try a cleanse – it may prove to be your fountain of youth.

WHAT TO AVOID WHILE DETOXING

First and foremost, avoid mercury in any fashion. Once you remove your mercury amalgams and your immune system starts dumping stored mercury, if you add mercury in any fashion you may have a violent reaction to the reintroduction of the poison. Avoid fish of all types and immunizations or allergy shots. Vaccines and allergy shots contain a preservative or antibacterial called thimersol. Thimersol contains mercury, which is the preservative used to kill bacteria in the serum. Until the medical profession can find an alternative to putting poison in shots it is best to avoid these even if healthy.

It is also important to avoid chemicals, paint, and perfumes, assuming you are not already sensitive to them. This means a change in life style, but a good health food store will have shampoos, conditioners, and soaps that are fragrance free. Many manufacturers make fragrance free detergents, and laundry products. Avoid all petrochemicals. If you heat with natural gas, consider changing to electricity, the hydrocarbons released by natural gas pose problems for many chemically sensitive individuals.

You should avoid foods that contain sugar or yeast. Alcohol should not be consumed in any fashion. If certain foods cause gastro problems avoid them and try to determine what ingredients in them create the problem. All dairy products should be eliminated with the possible exception of yogurt. Try yogurt and see if it settles OK. Eat only organic vegetables if possible and enjoy eggs. Eggs contain every amino acid and are one of the healthiest foods you can eat. In order for mercury to be excreted it is mandatory to have sufficient dietary fat. Fat transports mercury to the liver for excretion through bile. Hal Huggins, one of the pioneers in mercury detoxification recommends a stick of butter and three eggs everyday to help transport mercury for elimination. Additionally, don't forget the essential fatty acids mentioned previously.

Finally and most important, avoid or terminate relationships that are detrimental to your recovery. If you have determined that mercury is the cause of your illness and tests confirm it and you do not have support that is encouraging, you may never recover. This is the toughest battle you will ever encounter. The illness is not recognized by main street medicine, there is no traditional treatment, recovery and time of recovery is unpredictable, and the cost demands a change in life style. You will need support, and assistance in managing day to day activities. You will test the real meaning of love and commitment. Friends and loved ones who are supportive and understanding are critical to your successful recovery. Destructive relationships should be ended because they drain energy and you can only focus on one aspect of life: your recovery. The only casualty in your crusade is you, if others claim to be victims they are simply selfish uncaring individuals. The essence of love can be defined as sacrifice. If individuals who claim to love you are unwilling to sacrifice so you can regain your health you need to seriously question the relationship. You need to eliminate from your life those individuals that treat you with belligerence, abuse, and punish you because of your illness.

A recent study stated that couples that reported bad or unhappy marriages had more cavities than happily married people. It is comical to suggest dental hygiene is the road to a happy marriage. The message lost in the study is that mercury amalgams create neurological problems that severely test any relationships, including marriages.

If your doctor has a number of mercury toxic patients, try forming a support group and meet as often as you can to share success stories. Share books that others have bought, and articles that have been clipped. Determine what web sites have value and find chat groups that cater to sharing success stories regarding amalgam issues.

If possible, form a vitamin buying co-op group. It can save lots of money and is worth investigating. Compare the best vitamin prices you can get to the products offered on **www.thegreatdentaldeception.com**. Using the internet for information is worthwhile, but be aware that there are nuts dispensing information so filter out the good from the bad. I can assure you that some of the internet experts are quacks and are more dangerous than the mercury you are trying to eliminate.

Surround yourself with people that care about you, and are willing to help you. As you start feeling better become a resource for others, either in time, attention, information or access.

Studies state that people with positive attitudes increase their life expectancy by 7.5 years. Choose to be positive and don't let yourself become a victim. A positive approach helps you recover from illness and once recovered it extends your life.

The four principals of recovery:

.. DON'T BELIEVE TRADITIONAL MD'S. They are wrong.
.. DETOXIFYING FROM MERCURY IS A PROCESS, NOT AN EVENT. It takes time, in some cases years.
.. LEARN EVERYTHING YOU CAN FROM THIS BOOK AND OTHER SOURCES OF INFORMATION. Become an expert.
.. DON'T GIVE UP. Stay with the process of detoxification. You will see improvement eventually.

CHAPTER 9

Who Is Wise And Understanding Among You? Let Him
Show It By His Good Life, By Deeds Done In The
Humility That Comes From Wisdom.

THE ADRENALS, THE THYROID, AND MERCURY'S EFFECT

The adrenal glands are attached to the kidneys. The adrenal gland and the thyroid are responsible for producing energy. They release simple sugars, which serve as fuel for the body. The thyroid and the adrenals are frequently compromised when mercury is present. The effect is a loss of efficiency, and the result is a loss of energy or the symptom of fatigue.

The primary steroids produced by the adrenals are DHEA and cortisol. Cortisol is produced by the adrenals and is regulated by ACTH, a hormone produced by the pituitary gland (located in your brain).

Cortisol is established by the sleep/wake cycle, peaks in the morning and slowly decreases at night. It has a plethora of functions. One is response to stress, either physical or psychological. The stressor provokes cortisol to release as a mechanism to combat the problem. Mercury is a significant stressor. The increased levels of cortisol continue for a significant period of time until either the adrenals become exhausted or the stressor disappears. Other stressors are; infections, emotional stress, any toxin or a diet that is rich in sugar, carbohydrates, caffeine, and low in protein.

The typical adrenal response to mercury is elevated cortisol, followed in months or even years of very low levels. Another common trend is for low cortisol until evening, then it spikes. This is often an indication of a bacterial or viral infection. Measuring cortisol levels is easy. Many laboratories can determine cortisol levels simply by soaking cotton swabs in saliva. It is not an expensive test and provides critical information. This is done four times per day at specified times and then sent to the laboratory. If levels are low, prescribing hydrocortisone (cortisol) under the trade name cortef is potentially valuable. Dr. Jefferies's *Safe Uses of Cortisol* is well worth the read if you are concerned with taking cortisol.

Cortisol is very safe. Exhausted adrenals equal fatigue. Taking five mgs 1-4 times per day greatly benefits immune response, reduces fatigue, produces newfound energy and creates a sense of well-being. Dosages greater than five mgs can be prescribed but it is important to use cortisol under a doctor's supervision.

Adrenal fatigue can be one of the underlying causes of fibromyalgia, CFS, diabetes, allergies, anxiety, depression, liver dysfunction memory problems, being easily irritated and/or frustrated, as well as insomnia. Some additional symptoms that suggest adrenal problems are salt cravings, low HCL, hypoglycemia, loss of appetite, environmental sensitivities, muscle aches and pains, and food cravings. Mercury, the stressor, eventually creates adrenal exhaustion, and the lack of cortisol creates the symptoms mentioned above. Taking cortisol provides a sense of well-being. The goal is, however, to use cortisol on a temporary basis only. Reducing mercury levels allows the adrenals to produce adequate levels of cortisol and thus the reason to supplement is no longer necessary. Cortisol has a plethora of functions but it helps regulate blood sugar and is a strong anti-inflammatory.

In addition to cortisol, many practitioners substitute adrenal extract to supplement adrenal activity. The theory is that the extract supports adrenal activity while cortisol shuts down the adrenal production of cortisol. There is very little literature to support this conclusion and in Jeffries book, he states the opposite. He states that cortisol supplementation supports the adrenal production of cortisol and therefore provides the best support available. Needless to say, cortisol in whatever form provides benefits. The extract provides some cortisol since it is an extract. It is commonly agreed that the liquid adrenal extract is better than the tablet. However, the liquid is very expensive and is probably not necessary except in severe cases of adrenal exhaustion. Taking 6-12 tablets of adrenal extract per day is the recommended dosage for most people. I would recommend using cortisol (cortef) initially and determine energy levels, and then try the extract. If you get the same benefit, switch to the extract, or drastically reduce the amount of cortisol and use a combination of extract and cortisol. One of the problems with extracts is the inconsistency of each dosage, but many report great results with both the liquid and tablets. If you take cortisol, discuss wearing a medalert bracelet with your doctor, and when eliminating cortisol do it slowly and under a doctor's supervision.

Glandulars help rebuild body chemistry (the concept is based on the homeopathic theory that like cures like). For instance, a small amount of adrenal extract provides support for the adrenal gland, which promotes regeneration. It modulates cellular activity and supports a weakened gland. Glandulars are powerful tools that can assist the recovery of damaged glands. Glandular extracts, such as thyroid, pituitary, adrenal, spleen, pancreas, liver and thymus should be considered.

One way to measure adrenal function as you try combinations of cortisol and glandular extract is to take your blood pressure. Blood pressure is an excellent indicator of adrenal function. Low blood pressure signals tired adrenal glands, optimal blood pressure is 120/70. A number approximating this level means adrenal function is adequate and your supplementation program is working. However, blood pressure readings are only an indicator of adrenal efficiency. It is best to repeat the adrenal saliva test every 3-6 months.

Another test to determine adrenal function is the sodium/magnesium ratio from hair analysis. Take the mean number from the hair analysis for both minerals. Thus if the hair analysis states sodium should be between 5 and 15, the mean number is 10. Do this for both sodium and magnesium and develop an optimum ratio. Now use your actual numbers and see how close this number is to the optimum ratio you developed. If it is off by more than 7.5% your adrenals are not functioning properly and you are losing energy, and that creates symptoms of fatigue. The reason for using sodium and magnesium is that they are the two most important elements that comprise the adrenals. In all probability both are low, and the difference is far greater than 7.5%. In order to eliminate cortisol or the glandular extract, you must manage your body chemistry toward the optimum number. In all probability it means increasing your salt consumption and as stated in the supplement section, taking magnesium glycinate. Other supplements that help rebuild adrenals are significant amounts of vitamin C (10 grams or more spread throughout the day) garlic, chromium, alpha lipoic acid, essential fatty acids, and the amino acids taurine and tyrosine.

If you have any type of infection, mycoplasma or other pathogenic organisms then adequate levels of cortisol are mandatory in order to combat the infection. Absent sufficient quantities of cortisol the infection will proliferate regardless of the amount of antibiotics, herbs or other protocols that are used.

If you have adrenal exhaustion, then it is also probable that your DHEA is also low. DHEA regulates sex hormones and protects against many conditions associated with aging. Low DHEA is associated with aging. In addition low DHEA has been connected with hypertension, heart disease, diabetes, cancer, Lupus, and Alzheimers. In fact, most autoimmune diseases correlate with low DHEA levels.

DHEA, similar to cortisol, enhances the sense of well being. If DHEA is low men should take 10-20 mgs in the morning and females up to 5-0 mgs. If there is an exaggerated response to DHEA, then it is probably caused by a sulfation problem, identified in the liver detox section. If sulfation is low, supplementation with potassium and sodium sulfate, in an equal ratio, improves the sulfation pathway and provides a mechanism for DHEA to be appropriately used. If any of the detox panels in the liver test show a problem, be careful with DHEA supplementation. This could include phase one, phase two, methylation or sulfation. In some cases, DHEA supplementation can exaggerate the symptoms you are trying to improve. If this occurs stop using DHEA, until you resolve the detoxification pathways. Cortisol and DHEA work synergistically. So supplementation should be under a doctor's supervision.

The thyroid is another endocrine gland. One of its functions is to regulate metabolism (energy) and any inefficiencies in thyroid function effects every cell in a person's body. There are a number of tests that accurately access thyroid function. The best is a thyroid saliva test. Saliva tests are excellent tools for analyzing endocrine function since they evaluate what is available to cells. Traditional blood tests only evaluate what is floating around in the blood, not an accurate analysis at the cellular level. However, some of the more advanced thyroid blood tests provide excellent information on thyroid health. But in order to save money the saliva test is a good diagnostic tool. Some practitioners use both the blood and the saliva test as the most accurate methodology to analyze thyroid function. In addition to the saliva test take your temperature first thing in the morning, before you even get out of bed. Have a thermometer at your bedside and when you wake up immediately take your temperature. It can be done in two ways: your oral temperature – should be 98.2 degrees or above, your basal temperature, which is taken under your arm should be 97.8 degrees. Within two hours of waking, your oral temperature should be 98.6 degrees and remain there until bedtime. If any of your temperatures are below these numbers your thyroid is under stress.

Another excellent indicator of thyroid problems is elevated cholesterol, both total serum cholesterol, LDL and low HDL. Although most traditional doctors do not agree with this conclusion, evidence suggests cholesterol is an endocrine problem, not an eating disorder. If you have high cholesterol, then it is a good bet that you also have low temperatures in the morning. Finally low zinc guarantees a malfunctioning thyroid.

The thyroid produces a hormone: T4. This converted primarily by tissues as well as the liver into its active form T3. Most doctors prescribes a synthetic T4 for all conditions and then do follow up tests and temperature evaluations. In addition they ask you to monitor symptoms. Most of the time this is not be the solution. If T4 levels are adequate and T3 levels are low, then the body is not properly converting T4 to T3. (Often times adding B12 will solve the problem.) The solution might be a natural T3 product or a time released T3 supplement. In most mercury toxic individuals, TSH is high, free T4 can be all over the place and free T3 is low. Producing additional T3 is the key to providing relief to many symptoms that are caused by a malfunctioning thyroid. Many practitioners will prescribe a time released T3 that is ramped up until a temperature of 98.6 degrees is obtained and then gradually reduce the dosage with the hope that the thyroid will "kick in". This is called Wilson's Syndrome (not to be confused in any fashion with Wilson's Disease). This will not work. Do not waste your time or energy trying it. The solution is producing T3 consistently, not trying to spook your thyroid into producing it by hitting the correct level necessary to reach a temperature of 98.6 degrees and then slowly decreasing the amount of T3 in hopes of maintaining that level. The best solution is either a natural thyroid glandular that has a small amount of T4 and T3, or in finding a dosage of just enough T3 that produces a temperature of 98.6 degrees. In some cases individuals have an aberrant reaction to any amount of T4. This is due too a congested liver or inadequate levels of B12. In this case, the solution is a consistent time released T3 along with liver detoxification program, and B12 shots. Remember T4 is inactive and inert. The need is to create T3. The conversion of T4 to T3 requires selenium. If your hair analysis shows low selenium and thyroid function is abnormal, supplement 100 mcgs of selenium per day. Low selenium is very common in many mercury toxic individuals.

The reasons for thyroid problems are numerous. Examples include blood sugar problems due to carbohydrate addiction and a low protein diet.

Drugs such as antacids, antidepressants, aspirin, and beta blockers cause the thyroid to malfunction. Finally toxins such as mercury, lead, aluminum, radiation and contaminated water compromise thyroid health. All of these interfere with a thyroid's ability to function properly. Symptoms that correlate with a low body temperature (thyroid problems) are moodiness, low energy, fatigue, depression, dry skin, joint aches, weight gain, low blood pressure, high cholesterol, frequent infections, digestive, and sleeping problems, and libido problems. The other aspect of a low temperature is that enzymes are activated at various temperatures. If body temperatures are low, then many enzyme functions are inactivated throughout the entire body. It is critical to try and maintain a consistent body temperature of 98.6 degrees.

In addition to some form of T3 supplementation, DMPS injections directly into the thyroid are often valuable in chelating mercury from this important gland. Since T4 is primarily converted to T3 in the liver, a liver detoxification program is important. This should include a liver cleanse. In addition, be sure that you are getting enough iodine since this mineral is critical to the health of the thyroid.

As mentioned the thyroid secretes hormones that regulate metabolism in every cell in the body. In a healthy thyroid two tyrosine (an amino acid) molecules with two atoms of iodine create T4 (contains 4 molecules of iodine). This is regulated by the pituitary gland and its production of another hormone TSH. This creates a feedback system between the thyroid gland the pituitary gland. The problem with T4 and T3 production is typically in the thyroid process not the pituitary function. Typically the iodine molecules are compromised by mercury.

The thyroid has four binding sites for iodine. Mercury has a strong affinity for iodine, once mercury compromises one or more binding sites meant for iodine, then the thyroid cannot release the same quantity or quality of hormones it could before the presence of mercury. If your hair analysis shows below normal levels of iodine, supplement directly with iodine. This should be done under the direction of a doctor. The interesting aspect of iodine is that the Japanese consume about 30 times the RDA and have almost no thyroid problems. Be careful with the supplementation of iodine but it is critical to the proper functioning of the thyroid.

ENZYMES – ANOTHER IMPORTANT CHEMICAL ACTIVITY

Enzymes are needed for every chemical activity that occurs in the human body. Without enzymes, eating food causes stress on the entire endocrine system. Foods without enzymes also negatively affect blood sugar. Assuming you are eating wholesome foods, enzymes need a body temperature of 98.6 degrees to activate as well as the proper pH to be effective. If your temperature is not 98.6 degrees the enzymes are either deactivated or denatured. The chemical action is aborted; vitamins and minerals do not work without properly activated enzymes.

Enzymes are actually unique proteins. They aid digestion, deliver nutrients and enter the blood stream to assist the immune system in disposing of toxins.

HORMONES – ANOTHER VICTIM OF MERCURY'S INVASION

Hormones are powerful chemicals that influence our health. They affect our sense of well-being. Hormones are proteins that consist of amino acids; many of them consist of sulfur based amino acids. Mercury easily compromises those that contain SH groups, and once compromised the functionality of the hormone is altered. Glands produce hormones. The thyroid, pituitary and the adrenals are glands affected by mercury.

Since we have already discussed the thyroid and the adrenal glands in the previous section, this section focuses on the pituitary. The pituitary is located about two inches above the roof of your mouth. Mercury from mercury amalgams has easy access to this portion of the brain. The pituitary is considered a master gland. It sends messages to all the other glands, and when this master signal sender is rendered less than effective it impacts every hormone in our body. A Swedish study demonstrated that dentists have 800 times more mercury in their pituitary than non-dentists. Thus, let's assume that everyone with mercury amalgams has more mercury in their pituitary than people without mercury amalgams. Frequent urination and an overactive emotional state are symptoms that indicate a compromised pituitary. These are also indicators of mercury toxicity. This is not a coincidence. Detoxifying the pituitary is a challenge. The best option is DMSA. It crosses the blood brain barrier and pulls mercury from the brain.

The process of hormone production begins with the production of cholesterol. Total serum cholesterol produces pregnenalone, which then converts to DHEA and progesterone. The final conversion is testosterone and estrogen. Mercury affects the conversion process and the metabolism throughout the entire chain. It is very common for mercury toxic people to have elevated cholesterol and low hormones. This is simply an indicator that the conversion of cholesterol to hormones is compromised. Many practitioners offer hormone therapy that is a band-aid and provides a better quality of life, but like thyroid replacement, detoxifying allows nature to produce hormones naturally – that is the goal.

Mercury also interferes with glands responsible for sexual interest and reproduction capability. Typically the presence of mercury alters the following hormone pathways: estrogen, progesterone, and testosterone. The alteration in these hormones clearly explains the altered state of sexual interest. An interesting study concluded that when testosterone and estrogen are in balance serum phosphorous is also in balance.

Many practitioners believe the uterus is a collection center for mercury. Women who have long painful periods often resolve the problem with the removal of their mercury amalgams and undertaking the process of detoxification. Many times this only takes a few months. The process of a difficult period is nature's way of housecleaning and eliminating mercury. This fact certainly begs the question regarding the number of hysterectomies that are performed each year. Are they necessary? And if the uterus is simply the collection area for mercury where does the mercury go when the uterus is no longer in place and able to perform its function?

WHAT ROLE DOES pH PLAY IN MERCURY POISONING?

The pH of your system is critical for a successful recovery. Every medical doctor understands blood pH and, quite frankly, maintaining a neutral blood pH is necessary to live. Even the medical doctor who graduated last in his class understands this fact. Blood pH should be about 7.40. Most mercury patients are lower than 7.35 signifying an acidic condition. This seemingly small variance does not alarm most medical doctors since it is within the range set by most labs, however it is another variable in determining if you are mercury compromised. I recently met a patient who had a blood ph of 7.10. This is alarmingly low and signifies a serious problem.

The other part of pH is tissue or cellular pH, which is not understood or accepted by medical doctors. Every mercury patient I have met, who tested their tissue pH, has been acidic. This condition is called acidosis. However my sample is very small, thus I cannot conclude that every mercury patient has acidosis. When your body is overly acidic it has lost its alkaline reserve and many problems will occur. In the mercury toxic patient these problems are headaches, low blood pressure, foul smelling stools, a burning sensation in the anus, alternating constipation and diarrhea, and canker sores. Mercury is a cause of acidosis. Vitamin C can actually magnify an acidic condition, but citrus fruits actually help balance pH.

To test your pH purchase nitazine paper and urinate on a piece of this paper. Your packet will have a scale on it and depending what color develops will tell you if you are acidic. The ideal color equates to 7.2-7.5. If you are less than 7.0 consistently then you should take steps to balance your pH. If you can balance your pH to around 7.2 and thus actually create an alkaline condition you will feel much better and detoxify quicker. Most toxic people will actually have a pH less than 6.0.

My hypothesis is that you are acidic because you are mercury toxic. As long as you have high levels of mercury or other heavy metals in your system you will continue to have a low pH. As you chelate these toxins you should slowly see an improvement. Juicing or mixing any "green powder" is a great solution. This helps alkanize your system. Eating vegetables generally accomplishes the same thing but it will take much longer than some of the advertised "green drinks". Consume as many vegetables as you can per day. Try these combinations to see if you can alter your pH. Suffice to say most people agree you need to create an alkaline condition in order to detoxify.

Finally, when you are chelating with DMPS, check your pH a couple of times per day. In many cases DMPS will actually balance your pH. Only when you are through chelating will you need to reintroduce an alkaline product of some type. With frequent DMPS you may discover that your pH actually maintains a neutral position without any type of diet control. But this varies with all patients.

COPPER – A TRACE MINERAL OR A TOXIC HEAVY METAL?

One of the components of a mercury amalgam is copper. Copper is necessary in very small amounts for life. However, as part of the mercury amalgam copper is also released in the same way mercury is released and absorbed in the same fashion. Excess copper only accentuates mercury problems. The best indicator of copper levels is a hair analysis.

A number of indicators in the hair analysis indicate a copper burden. The obvious indicator is elevated copper; however there are a number of hidden indicators of copper excess. These include, high calcium, a zinc to copper ratio less than 6:1, sodium to potassium ratio less than 2.2:1, a calcium to potassium ratio greater than 10:1, and high mercury. All the above are potential indicators of high copper.

If copper is a serious problem, copper should be elevated and zinc will be low in the hair analysis and the hidden indicators will all demonstrate a copper problem. Copper and zinc are antagonists and should be kept in balance. When out of balance copper and zinc create two problems: excess copper is toxic and reduced zinc creates different problems. Zinc is involved in over 200 enzymatic functions and low zinc disrupts metabolic pathways involving zinc. Fixing the problem is complex. If copper is high then mercury is also probably very high. DMPS and DMSA chelate both copper and mercury. Taking zinc helps. Avoiding copper in all vitamins and avoiding high copper foods is important. Don't add to the burden, and be sure to increase zinc dosages after any chelating cycle. In addition, adequate adrenal function is necessary in order to lower copper levels.

Zinc metabolism is tied to cortisol availability, so if cortisol is low zinc does not absorb and copper will continue to win the battle of the two minerals. Increasing cortisol levels aids in the absorption of zinc and helps eliminate copper. The majority of copper is excreted in bile and a small percent is excreted in the urine, thus the need for proper liver function. Liver cleanses and liver detoxification protocol should be undertaken.

High levels of zinc supplementation can increase LDL, so be careful if using high levels of zinc for protracted periods of time. Typically, once mercury is eliminated and supplementation is appropriate, it takes at least a year to rebalance zinc and copper.

Often times the liver has problems detoxifying due to the relationship of copper to zinc. If the ratio in the hair analysis is less than 4:1, zinc to copper, the liver cannot detoxify effectively. In addition, protein digestion is impaired, which is one of the reasons why an amino acid profile is important. It identifies amino acid deficiencies that need to be corrected. The ratio that is optimal is 7.5:1, zinc to copper. As is probably obvious, the human body is a very complex structure. Everything is connected. It mystifies me how the era of specialization is an advantage to a patient.

Many times physicians see elevated copper and immediately diagnose Wilsons Disease. This is a rare disease that is characterized by the inability to metabolize copper. It is not a disease that manifests itself at age 40, but is a product of birth. Very few people have Wilsons Disease also test positive for mercury toxicity. It is simply copper excess from mercury amalgams.

In the 1970s a new amalgam mix was introduced that had similar amounts of mercury but the copper portion increased dramatically; the percentage of copper was between 26-33% of the mixture. Research on the amalgam mix suggests the new composition of metals causes mercury and copper to be released faster and at higher levels; in some studies the release of mercury increased by more than 50 times from the original amalgam. In addition, the copper released by the amalgam increased. This new mixture was labeled "state of the art" by the ADA (who had patents on the new mixture). Some speculate that this amalgam mixture is the reason for the increase in autoimmune diseases, Alzheimer's disease, and cancer. Also, the speculation is that the reason the average age autoimmune diseases are contracted is much lower than in the past is because of this amalgam mix.

It is interesting that studies illustrate that gold placed in the vicinity of a mercury amalgam restoration produces a ten-fold increase in the release of mercury. This is just speculation but imagine the toxicity of a gold crown on the surface, and a high copper amalgam below it. Sounds like lots of mercury and copper are released and absorbed.

Elevated copper levels reduce histamine levels. Histamine is commonly associated with allergies. But it is also a critical neurotransmitter and influences behavior. Low histamine creates an overabundance of methyl groups (over methylation) and thus excessive levels of dopamine and other important neurotransmitters. This condition is called histapenia. It may be a genetic function or the condition might result from excess toxins. It magnifies an already dangerous situation. Mercury by itself creates all types of neurological problems but add to that a huge amount of cooper which results in low histamine and all types of behavioral problems can occur. And usually do. Histapenia can be confirmed with a blood test. A few indicators that correlate to low histamine; high copper levels and low zinc levels in the hair analysis, a low sex drive, anxiety, trouble getting to sleep at night, and trouble waking up in the morning, food and chemical sensitivities, lots of dental decay, and depression. Supplements that must be avoided are methionine in any form, glycine, tryptophan, tyrosine, any form of garlic supplement, DMSA, and MSM; these all effect methylation and this is already too high. If you use these supplements and get an aberrant reaction stop using them immediately and suspect histapenia. Also do not use Prozac, Paxil, antacids or antihistamines such as Benadryl. Very useful supplements include folic acid, as much as 10 mgs per day, B6, niacin, and the most important B12. Most people benefit from B12 shots every day. There should be no concern regarding the toxicity of B12. It is a benign vitamin. But watch cobalt levels on your hair analysis. Depending on the strength of the B12 that you are administering a couple of cc's can provide an incredible change in your health in only a few days. If this condition has caused mental illness it may take up to a year to correct. No drug will work, only the vitamins mentioned above. It is also possible that mercury toxic people can have high histamine levels. In this case the opposite applies. Methionine, glycine et al will have a positive influence while B12 etc will have a negative impact. **Histamine levels will greatly affect the traditional detoxification protocols that doctors recommend in eliminating mercury from your body. It is always overlooked by every doctor treating mercury burden. And it is critical information to understand.** In some cases high copper levels will marginally decrease histamine levels but they are still well within the reference range. However many of the above symptoms will appear and the protocol to eliminate the symptoms are the same. When copper levels are reduced the need for B12 etc often times disappears.

A couple of interesting studies relating to copper deserve mention. One study demonstrated high copper levels in fingernails of infants with cystic fibrosis, the other that diabetes is due to the interference of copper with zinc and therefore affects glucose metabolism.

In detoxifying from copper excess, often copper is mobilized from tissue faster than it can be excreted. This is often referred to as a copper dump (a healing event). Symptoms include nausea, itching, a rash, fatigue, aches

117

and pains, chills, nervousness, insomnia, and gastro intestinal problems. The result is frequent liver releases. This is determined by looking in the toilet and a thick yellow liquid is visible. These symptoms can last up to 48 hours. It feels like you have the flu, but it is not. It is not contagious. It is your body, via the liver excreting copper as well as other toxins. Believe it or not, this is a great sign.

The greater the number of healing events a person experiences, the faster the road to recovery. However, it is important to prepare mentally for these events. It can be discouraging unless you are aware that it is a healing event. Remember healing events are eliminating a toxin that is impeding your road to recovery.

If your child's hair analysis shows elevated copper and low zinc contact the Pheiffer Clinic. The facility is in Naperville, Illinois and named after a pioneer in copper toxicity, Dr. Carl Pheiffer. The clinic specializes in learning disabilities in children due to copper excess. It is the clinic's belief that learning disabilities are often times a result of impaired body chemistries, particularly copper. Balance the body chemistries and the disabilities disappear. My experience is that they are very good with young people, but their success with adults is not as good. They attempt to correct chemical imbalances with vitamins and this can be successful in young people. The older the person is, more is required than simple supplementation. But their diagnosis is invaluable.

In addition to the clinic in Naperville, they travel periodically to other parts of the country as part of an outreach program. The objective of the clinic is to resolve copper imbalances through the use of vitamins, minerals, and amino acids. Again, they seem to be most successful with children who have learning disabilities.

VACCINATIONS... HIDDEN MERCURY

"Vaccines are the only drugs that Americans are required by a government agency to take. The federal government is also the largest purchaser of vaccines. It is thus imperative that the federal government ensures the safety of these mandated vaccines." Quote by Representative Dan Burton, July 18, 2000

Most vaccinations contain thimersol, a mercury preservative, which acts as an antibacterial. It was introduced into vaccines in 1950. It is interesting to note the dramatic rise in ADD, autism, SIDS and various learning disabilities over the past 50 years. Many believe it is a direct result of mercury being added to vaccines. In other words, mercury is put into vaccines to protect the vaccine from viruses and bacteria. At one point there were over 50 vaccines that contained mercury.

The only vaccines that did not contain mercury were the live virus vaccines, for example measles and mumps. All others contain mercury, including hepatitis B, which is given to every new born at birth. Think about this, doctors inject a new born with a vaccine containing one of the most toxic substances on this planet when they are less than 48 hours old. This is a recipe for disaster, and disaster is just what we have created. All childhood maladies have increased during the last 50 years. Asthma is reaching epidemic proportions, juvenile diabetes is increasing every decade, autism, and A.D.D. are no longer rare in communities but common in most neighborhoods.

Dr. Boyd Haley at the University of Kentucky suggests an infant now has a variety of sources of mercury. As a fetus, elemental mercury from a pregnant mom's mercury amalgams passes through the placenta creating a tremendous toxic burden while in the womb, the mother's milk is contaminated with mercury from mercury amalgams and vaccines that an infant receives contain mercury. This is a huge burden for a 6-8 pound baby to eliminate this toxin when it has limited bile production and renal function at birth In addition the blood brain barrier is not fully developed in infants. Add to this the fact that some vaccines contain aluminum and formaldehyde and the poor infant is challenged to be healthy. It is a catastrophe waiting to happen.

Recently it was determined that babies who receive multiple vaccinations with thimersol exceed the EPA's limit on mercury. Typically, a newborn has six vaccinations in the first few months of life and 11 by their 2nd birthday. The quantum leap in the number of vaccines a child receives in their first 24 months of life guarantees they exceed the EPA's threshold for mercury. The reality is that the EPA's tolerance for mercury in children should be zero. The 1/2 life of mercury guarantees mercury builds up in all babies under two years old, and guarantees mercury resides in most children for a prolonged period of time. The concern is how much build up is too much. The answer is that no child should be exposed to a poison at any level. Particularly in a government mandated vaccine.

If you must get a vaccine insist on a new vial. Mercury as we have discussed is a heavy metal and concentrates on the bottom of a vial. Nurses are suppose to shake the vial prior to drawing the vaccine into the syringe, however if this does not occur the final few shots will contain higher levels of mercury. The extra blast of mercury might be all it takes to cause damage.

In reality the history of problems with thimersol in vaccines can be traced back to April 1930. Eli Lilly, a primary supplier of vaccinations, studied thimersol in patients known to be dying of meningococcal meningitis. This study and research is regarded as highly questionable, nevertheless Lilly cited their research for decades as proof that thimersol created minimal toxicity and was harmless to humans. Subsequent to the 1930 research, information that was contrary to the Lilly research should have caused all providers of thimersol vaccines to cease production immediately.

- In 1950 a *NY Academy of Science* article stated that mercury is toxic when ingested into anyone and should not be used in chemotherapy.
- In 1963 an article suggested that some people react to mercury that is ingested and for these people another preservative should be used.
- In 1967 it was requested that the claim "non toxic" that is used on thimersol labels be deleted in the next printing of warning labels.
- In 1967 the words non toxic are omitted and replaced with "non-irritating" to body tissues.
- In 1972 it is reported that mercury in vaccines caused six deaths.
- In 1976 Eli Lilly objected to warnings on thimersol products stating, "We are not aware of any instance of mercury poisoning after decades of marketing this product. This is because the mercury is organically bound and is completely non-toxic." (Sound familiar? Identical to an ADA position on amalgams.)
- In 1982 the FDA stated, "At the cellular level, thimersol has been found to be more toxic to human cells in vitro than mercuric chloride..."(and other forms of mercury).
- In 1983 Lilly adds the following warning to thimersol labels: "If you are pregnant or nursing, seek the advice of a health professional before using this product."
- In 1999 MSDS warnings regarding thimersol,
  1) Mercury poisoning may occur
  2) Exposure in children may cause mild to severe retardation

3)   Hypersensitivity, to mercury, is a medical condition aggravated by exposure.

To summarize thimersol used in vaccines has been dangerous since its introduction. Increased usage has increased symptoms and the severity of each symptom. Similar to the ADA, vaccine manufacturers were aware of the dangers and rationalized their usage for profits. Kids have died, suffered disease and neurological symptoms because of this indifference.

Sounds like the MSDS on thimersol should be discussed with all parents before vaccines are given to their precious child. No informed consent exists between pediatricians and parents – this is criminal.

Recently the *Journal of the American Medical Association* published a study stating the measles, mumps, and rubella vaccine could, but not by itself, cause autism. The MMR vaccine does not contain mercury; the study only looked at that one vaccine. The study did not evaluate the total vaccine burden. Interestingly, a spokesman for the Autism Research Institute in San Diego says in spite of the study, the vaccine cannot be dismissed as a possible link to autism (The important word is link). The referenced study occurred between 1980 and 1994. Between 1980 and 1986 73% of the applicable population received the MMR shot, this number increased to 81% from 1988 to 1994. During this time period autism increased dramatically. Not studied but very relevant is that fact that the total number of vaccinations children received rose during this time period.

The spokesman for the Autism Institute stated further that it might be the number of vaccinations children get at once, rather than the MMR vaccine by itself. He continued by commenting that the mercury in most vaccines could "disable the immune system, so the kid's ability to handle the measles virus is greatly reduced." He suggested the relationship between autism and vaccines requires additional research. More and more research is beginning to connect the increase in vaccinations to the epidemic increase in autism.

Unfortunately the following scenario could endanger a child, he/she is given a typical round of vaccinations during his/her first two months of life, and the impact is the child receives 62.5 micrograms of mercury or 125 times the EPA's limit. This is a huge burden of mercury and clearly poses a potentially impossible challenge for a young immune system. The child is later diagnosed with a mild form of autism or ADD. This is a common occurrence in our society.

A number of class action lawsuits have been filed against vaccine manufacturers. For additional information visit the web site www.vaccineinjury.org if you feel someone you know was harmed by vaccines. It is worth investigating your options. Very intelligent people that understand the toxic effects of mercury made a conscious decision to place mercury in vaccines that are given to infants with reckless abandon. This seems to be criminal.

Surgeon General David Satcher, recently issued the following statement, "The risk of devastating diseases from failure to vaccinate far outweighs the minimal, if any, risk of exposure to cumulative levels of mercury in vaccines." This is unbelievable. Our Surgeon General recognizes the cumulative effects of mercury in newborns and minimizes the effect. I surmise he has never been affected by the news that a child has ADD, died of SIDS, or is impacted by asthma or juvenile diabetes.

The good news is that the pediatric associations are asking manufacturers to eliminate thimersol from all vaccines. As of the publication of this book, many manufacturers are researching ways to produce vaccines without mercury. The tremendous challenge for concerned parents is to find a way to get the benefit of vaccinations without the dire effects of mercury. The challenge is made even more difficult since vaccines are the only drugs that are mandated by the federal government. The federal government is thus legislating every precious newborn must receive high levels of mercury in vaccinations.

Some allergy shots and flu shots also contain thimersol. No child under any circumstances should get a flu shot. The extra dose of mercury is not worth the trade off. Mercury burden or the possibility of getting the flu, the only bet to make as a parent is the potential to get the flu for a few days. Allergy shots should be avoided by anyone who is trying to detoxify from mercury. In reality allergy shots should be replaced by other methods. A weekly blast of mercury does not seem to make sense for anyone.

WHY DO I NEED TO KNOW ALL THIS?

So far, I have given you an enormous amount of information regarding mercury, the effects it has on the human body, and methods to excrete it from various organs. The obvious question is if a patient has all this knowledge, doctors must know even more and therefore I should be able to depend on a doctor, particularly if that doctor is an alternative physician. Hopefully, someday that might be true. Today it is not true, it is unlikely that you will be lucky enough to find any type of doctor that has the information contained in this book. You must become responsible for your own health.

A few comments from doctors that I saw will convince you that you must become an expert regarding mercury. The alternative is to depend on doctors who made the following comments:

Gastro Dr. #1 – There is no reason for the symptoms you are experiencing. We have done every test imaginable. I suggest you see a different doctor.

Gastro Dr #2 – Unless you have some strange disease from Africa there is nothing physically wrong with you. You need to see a shrink.

Shrink – I have no idea what's causing all the symptoms. I'm going to prescribe a antidepressant drug even though you exhibit no signs of depression.

Naturopathic Dr. #1 – You are allergic to every food substance. I can desensitize you and make you well for about $10,000.

Environmental Dr. #1 – The rash caused by the DMPS challenge concerns me (this is a common side effect) thus I do not want to treat you any longer. Plus your mercury levels are so high I think its best to find another doctor.

Homeopathic Dr. #1 – In order to eliminate mercury I need to prescribe small doses of mercury in order to mobilize your system to eliminate mercury.

Environmental Dr. #2 – The huge amounts of copper and the zinc deficiency suggest you need to take five mg of copper per day.

Naturopathic Dr. #2 – The cost of the test is $800.00 and we will be able to discuss the results telephonically. This is my specialty. I have patients all over the country that I work with over the telephone. (The tests were done and the guy never returned my calls, or correspondence.)

Large Immune Center in Southern California – I'm ordering a MRI on the pituitary, an ultrasound on the thyroid, a comprehensive blood panel and scheduling a telephone conference when the results come in. (I scheduled three different telephone conferences, waited four hours each time, no one called to cancel them or reschedule, eventually I took the test results to a different doctor.)

Dentist #1 – Mercury is perfectly safe. You are wasting your money. As a friend do not go down this road.

Oral surgeon #1 – Root canals are safe, I will not extract your tooth. I do four to six root canals a day and have for 20 years and if there was a problem I would know about it.

Talk show host – A popular syndicated medical talk show hosted by a medical doctor was discussing mercury amalgams with a caller and as expected the "expert" defended the mercury amalgam. This was no surprise. The proof statement was that according to him our body needs micro-doses of every element, including mercury. Thus, receiving minute amounts of mercury from our mercury amalgams is good news and we are healthier because mercury amalgams are releasing mercury vapor. This was his argument. I tried desperately to call him and ask if he would support a "multi-vitamin" that contained not only mercury, but also arsenic, lead, plutonium, cadmium, tin, and aluminum in it. If every element has some value to human health then just to be sure we are receiving appropriate amounts we need this new "multi-vitamin." He could endorse it. His call screener would not let me through to talk to him. But I bet many listeners no longer fear heavy metals due to his utterly stupid comment.

Environmental Doctor #2 – Five years ago I would have made a preliminary diagnosis of M.S based on the visual symptoms, and early onset AD based on the severe memory loss. I would have followed up with testing to confirm or rule out my diagnosis. Today, I agree you should focus on mercury removal and determine which of these symptoms improve.

The above are true statements made by licensed doctors. Unfortunately, I followed some of the suggestions, which is my fault and only lengthened the time it took to get my health back. If I knew then what I know now, the time it took to regain my health would have been cut in half. In spite of all the bad experiences I was fortunate to find one terrific doctor and together we found answers. I was also lucky to find a great oral surgeon for cavitation work (discussed later in the book). As you can tell from some of the above comments, there are some very heartless doctors who prey on the hopeless and sick, and try to make a quick buck. This is one of the really sad facts I discovered on my journey toward health.

As my health returned I wrote all the allopathic and other doctors and informed them of my return to health and hoped they would consider mercury from amalgams as a health hazard. I felt compelled to provide this information, and I did not expect any responses. The mainstream doctors never mentioned amalgams to me while I was searching for answers, and I assumed my letter was a waste of time. But I had information and maybe just one of them would read it. Surprisingly, I did get one letter back. Gastro Dr. #2, a highly respected doctor in the area, thanked me for the letter, stated he already had begun the process of having his amalgams removed and planned on expediting the process based on my letter. I appreciated the letter, but think about it. He already knew of the dangers of mercury in amalgams, was having his replaced but did not want to rock the boat by practicing what he believed in. The AMA must be a very intimidating organization. You probably will discover that you will work with multiple doctors in order to regain your health. One doctor might have expertise in DMPS but not have experience with thyroid problems and the value of T3. A different doctor could be an expert in infections. Don't be leered into using only one doctor. Take advantage of each doctors expertise.

The message is that you must be informed. Read everything you can get your hands on, become another mercury expert.

Recovery is based on the following four principles:

.. **DON'T BELIEVE TRADIONAL MDs REGARDING MERCURY. They are wrong.**
.. **DETOXING FROM MERCURY IS A PROCESS, NOT AN EVENT. It takes time, in some cases years.**
.. **LEARN EVERYTHING YOU CAN FROM THIS BOOK AND OTHER SOURCES OF INFORMATION. Become an expert.**
.. **DON'T GIVE UP. Stay with the process of detoxing. You will see improvement eventually.**

CHAPTER 10

HE GIVES WISDOM TO THE WISE AND KNOWLEDGE TO THE DISCERNING

ALZHEIMER'S DISEASE (A.D)

Tom Warren's *Beating Alzheimer's* is a must read for everyone. This book describes the journey of the author from an A.D diagnosis to its successful remission. The cure for him was removing all his mercury amalgams, having cavitation surgery, detoxifying with DMPS, and supplementing with vitamins and minerals. The book proves there is at least one cure for A.D. It is the removal of dental amalgams. In addition to reading the book visit a very convincing web site: www.testfoundation.org/admercury.htm

A.D was first described in medical literature in 1838. Remember, the mercury amalgam was introduced to Europe in 1820 and to the United States in 1833. The introduction of the mercury amalgam and the first report of A.D are only a few years apart. It is important to understand that A.D manifests itself at various rates. An important fact to understand: toxins are fat soluble. Our body stores toxins in fatty tissues and the human brain is approximately 70% fat. Thus the human brain is contaminated with a plethora of toxins including mercury.

In a Canadian research project rats inhaled mercury vapor four hours per day for two weeks. The amount of mercury vapor was approximately equal to the amount of vapor released by mercury amalgams. Upon autopsy, the rat's brain exhibited the traditional tangles and plaques that are characteristic in A.D. Although literature described the malady in 1838 it was not named or "discovered" until 1906 by German doctor Alois Alzheimer. He announced his discovery of a disease of the cerebral cortex. Plaques and tangles that inhibit brain functions mark the disease. This is exactly the same description that Canadian research described in mercury toxic rats.

In autopsy studies of A.D victims zinc and selenium are significantly below normal. These two minerals are also deficient in mercury toxic patients. And both are often recommended as supplements in a mercury detoxification program. This is a fascinating relationship.

Separate research conducted between 1997 and 2000 by Olivieri, Prendergrass, and Haley, all concluded that mercury from mercury amalgams are toxic to human brain cells and cause the formation of amyloid plaques, and neuro-fibrillan tangles in tissue cultures. These are common characteristics of Alzheimer's.

A Massachusetts General Hospital study in 2001 suggests a build up of copper in the brain causes protein deposits that are the hallmarks of A.D. The neuro-fibrillan tangles of amyloid plaques traps copper in its tangles, this causes oxygen and hydrogen to form hydrogen peroxide – a cell toxin just like mercury. What could cause excess copper? One possible cause is reduced zinc due to mercury's effect on the zinc/copper relationship, and therefore excess copper. Another is the release of copper from high copper mercury amalgams and this excess copper has easy access to the brain.

Autopsies demonstrate up to four times more mercury in an A.D brain than a non-A.D brain. Where did this mercury come from? The most obvious source is mercury amalgams. Daily environmental exposure cannot produce this quantity of mercury. And remember mercury is a serious neurotoxin. It's hard to fathom anything that could cause more damage to the brain than mercury.

The hippocampus is an area of the brain that contains one of the largest concentrations of metals in the body – both good and bad metals. For instance, it contains zinc and copper in high amounts, and attracts dangerous metals such as aluminum and mercury. Although the dangers of mercury and aluminum in the hippocampus are obvious, the dangers of inappropriate levels of copper and zinc are equally as dangerous. The hippocampus is an area of the brain that is responsible for memory, learning and behavior control. Typically an A.D sufferer has problems in all three of these areas.

A.D is currently growing at a rapid rate. We need to understand that mercury is released from amalgams over decades at a slow rate. It is absorbed in the brain. The blood brain barrier is ineffective in keeping mercury from entering the brain. Mercury is building progressively in the brain. Mercury kills all living cells. We are seeing A.D diagnosed at younger and younger ages. Based on the volume of mercury in the average mouth the amazing fact is that more people are not diagnosed with A.D. and it is quite possible that if we keep using 100 tons of mercury every year in the dental profession, the estimates predicting the growth of A.D might be conservative.

Dr. Boyd Haley, Chair of the Chemistry Department at the University of Kentucky, has done extensive research on the connection between A.D and mercury amalgams. He believes there is a possible relationship between A.D and the mercury released from dental amalgams. One of the symptoms that exists in A.D is that both beta-tubulin and cratine kinase are significantly reduced in the brain of A.D sufferers (Various autopsies show the brain of a person not diagnosed with A.D has 2000% more cratine kinase than a person with A.D). Haley did experiments and concluded that adding mercury vapor to a non-A.D brain would cause the reduction of these two proteins in a healthy brain. Again mercury amalgams are the only logical source of mercury. All the pieces exist for this to be a primary cause of A.D, a poison that has proximity to the brain, and that has the ability to cause cell damage.

At this point, no research has suggested A.D is genetic. Nor can it be explained by environmental data. Statistically A.D is similar state to state, and rural versus urban. The conclusion that is generated is that a person must be exposed to something to get A.D. Scientists want us to believe it is genetic in spite of evidence to the contrary, since it supports the growth of the disease, but nothing supports the genetic theory. In other words, if my grandfather had A.D and my dad had it then I am at serious risk. The simple truth is that science does not specifically support this hypothesis. Science does support a detoxification gene but in all probability the better question is did they both have mercury amalgams?

A small group of researchers, including Haley, believe the reason everyone with mercury amalgams does not have A.D is that certain blood proteins control cholesterol build up in the brain and assist in the elimination of mercury from the brain and other proteins cause its retention. Apoprotein (APOE) controls mercury detoxification in the brain. The molecular composition of APOE could be the underlying source of A.D pathology. The overall function of APOE is to remove cholesterol from the brain, however depending on the genetic make-up of the APOE gene it is also designed to transport mercury out of the brain along with excess cholesterol. The APOE2 gene has two cysteine molecules. Cysteine is a sulfur-based amino acid and research indicates individuals with this genotype rarely ever get A.D. APOE3 has one cysteine molecule and one arginine molecule. This genotype is moderately at risk for A.D. And the APOE4 genotype is comprised of two arginine molecules and people with this genotype are eight times more likely to be diagnosed with A.D than someone with APOE3. Thus the genetic link might exist but not based on traditional theories. The solution to overcome the predisposition to A.D (the APOE4 genotype) is to eliminate any mercury source and supplement with the sulfur-based amino acids. Great Smokies Laboratory now offers a test, which provides you with genetic testing, including the APOE genotype. It is expensive, but well worth the investment.

A genetic relationship might exist between the protein that helps cause detoxification and the protein that causes retention, but certainly it is not the death sentence suggested by A.D "experts." A.D research indicates that if your family has a history of A.D then you at a similar risk, and there is not much you can do about it. In order to reduce the risk of A.D, just have your mercury amalgams removed and detoxify your body. Then, regardless of the APOE gene you inherit your risk of A.D is reduced, if not eliminated, since the cause of the disease is eliminated. The concern for the genetic predisposition is now irrelevant since mercury no longer has access to the brain and thus the gene that creates retention is irrelevant.

Haley suggests that since mercury is such a powerful neurotoxin, and since mercury is released from mercury amalgams, then mercury amalgams are risky for anyone with neurological disease. These diseases would include A.D, Parkinson's, ALS and MS. If the cause and effect is not mercury amalgams, then mercury amalgams, at a minimum, increase the severity of these diseases.

A recent study compared the risk of A.D in a sample of African-American men in the United States and a group of men from a country in Africa. The outcome of the study was that the men in United States had twice the likelihood of getting A.D. The study concluded that diet must play a role in A.D. Further studies are planned to determine what role diet plays in the higher rate of A.D in the United States. This suggests that good nutrition causes A.D – this is truly comical. What should be studied is how did dental care compare? What group had the most mercury amalgams? Did either group have more root canals than the other? There is a real danger in prejudging the above information, but taking this risk, I think the African-Americans had more mercury amalgams, more root canals, and the sample in Africa had fewer teeth; thus fewer toxins in their mouth. But the research group did not even consider mercury, and instead decided to analyze diet.

The biggest challenge is not the risk of A.D, but finding a way to get the mercury out of your brain once you decide to get the source removed. Without a chelating agent you cannot remove mercury. You cannot live long enough to get rid of the mercury. So how do we remove mercury from the brain? The answer is using DMSA and alpha lipoic acid. These cross the blood brain barrier and transport mercury for elimination. If you believe neurological symptoms are a problem, these two medicines should be part of your protocol. Typical symptoms that suggest brain impairment are memory loss, anger, temper tantrums, depression, anxiety and insomnia. In addition take choline and lecithin; these are neurotransmitter precursors that provide nourishment to brain cells. Vitamin B12, B6, and folic acid are now being used by many traditional neurologists as part of the protocol to slow the progression of A.D. The dosages are not enough but it's a start. There are studies using these particular vitamins to access their impact on delaying or improving critical thinking and memory.

The only warning regarding DMSA is the good news is that it crosses the blood brain barrier, and the bad news is that it crosses the blood brain barrier. Early in your detox process you do not want any drug that crosses the barrier. Theoretically it could "pick up" mercury and transport it to the brain. Thus do not use DMSA until the majority of the mercury is eliminated from everything but your brain. Then it is safe to use DMSA as a chelator. The one thing you do not want to do is provide mercury access to the brain through a drug you think is moving mercury out of your system.

An expert at the 1997 National Vaccine Information Center Conference stated a person who received a flu shot in five consecutive years increased their risk of A.D ten times over someone who received no flu shots. It is amazing that we are still debating the damage thimersol causes in vaccines and flu shots.

Currently it is projected that over $1,000,000,000 was spent on memory enhancing drugs in the year 2002. In addition it is projected that total A.D medical costs will approximate $4,000,000,000 in the year 2002 and $14,000,000,000 by 2050. In my particular case, and most others that I know who have or had mercury problems, problems occur in both short term and long term memory. It was common for me to arrive at my ATM and have no clue what my code was. I forgot names; my day timer had everything from business responsibilities to vitamins that I needed to take. I simply had no memory function. Now, seven years after mercury amalgam removal, I no longer forget my ATM code, and rarely even use my day timer. I can tell you what my schedule looks like one month from now. I do not have the dramatic story Tom Warren tells in his book, but I overcame memory problems by having my mercury amalgams removed. Rather than spend billions on memory drugs, attack the cause with our money. Get the mercury out of your mouth.

Did you know the proximity of mercury in your tooth to your brain is less than one inch? We already know mercury is released. We also know that it is a powerful neurotoxin. Mercury has a negative effect on your brain and your brain's necessary functions. Do you need to be a medical doctor to come to a common sense conclusion? If you are concerned with potential neurological disease, then remove your mercury amalgams.

In India only 1% of the population suffers from A.D. In the United States 10% of those over 65 have the malady and 50% over 85 years of age have been diagnosed with A.D. Research is being performed to determine if tumeric reduces the risk of A.D. This is a common herb used in most Indian cooking. This is an inexpensive herb to take. Until this research is completed it is probably worth taking.

A.D is the fourth leading cause of death in the United States in people over 75, which is amazing for a disease that did not exist 150 years ago. Not surprisingly, it is growing at a faster rate than any other disease. It is time responsible research determines if the link between heavy metals, specifically mercury is a causative factor in A.D. Senior citizens should live their twilight years with an excellent quality of life and pride, not the humiliating effects that A.D causes.

CANCER

Various groups report up to 75% of all cancer might be caused by environmental toxins. For instance, in 1992 United States companies released almost two billion pounds of toxic chemicals into the air. The air quality in L.A. creates a 450 times greater probability of cancer, based on standards established by the Federal Clean Air Act, than cities in other parts of the country. Any toxin damages the cell membrane and cellular

DNA. This provides the opportunity for malignancy throughout the body. The cause can be debated, but the fact is that 25% of all deaths in the year 2000 were from cancer as opposed to 3% in 1900.

The relationship between cancer and mercury amalgams deserves serious research. In Dr. Hassen's *The Prevention and Cure of Cancer*, Dr. Hassen states unequivocally that most all the cancer he has treated was preceded by inflammation in the root of a tooth. Other doctors and clinics state that **all** cancer patients are heavy metal toxic, either lead, aluminum, or mercury, with particular focus on mercury. We know mercury causes all of the following: promotes free radical production, hinders DNA repair, and reduces glutathione. Each of these causes have been linked to factors increasing the probability of cancer.

Every hypothesis states that cancer can be seriously mitigated if a consumer attempts to control the environment he/she lives in.

BREAST CANCER

There have been no studies regarding the relationship between breast cancer and mercury amalgams, but there are some very strong correlations:

1. Many studies have demonstrated mercury in high concentrations is found in mother's milk. This mercury toxic milk is passed to infants and studies indicate there is a relationship between toxic milk and SIDS, leukemia, and A.D.D. in the children. Certain studies suggest women who breast-feed are at less risk of breast cancer. Is it because they have detoxified the toxins out of their breasts and into their babies?

2. Breasts are in close proximity to the lungs and the lungs are the initial pathway mercury takes when it is released from the amalgam.

3. A study published in 1989 reported a high incidence of breast cancer in women who suffered from constipation. Constipation is a common symptom of mercury toxicity. Slow bowel transit time has also been linked to colon cancer. Colon cancer kills 50000 Americans each year, and is the second most common form of cancer. A Chinese proverb states that large frequent stools equal small hospitals. It is very clear that constipation, and infrequent bowel movements allow

toxins to build up. Increasing fiber is critical to good health and reducing the odds of getting any type of cancer.

The above facts suggest that as opposed to the phrase, Race for The Cure, the real grassroots effort should focus on the "Race for Prevention." The millions of dollars that courageous women raise to combat this horrible disease should focus on the cause, not drugs to treat breast cancer once it invades the body. It seems based on the impact mercury has on our immune system this would be a good place to spend some research money. There is certainly enough circumstantial evidence to suggest a relationship.

The increase in the propensity for a female to contract breast cancer is alarming. In 1961 the incidence of breast cancer was 1 in 20, in 1994 1 in 8, and in 2000 it was 1 in 5. Something has caused this dramatic increase and the reason needs to be determined before every woman must face this horrible disease.

To provide creditability to the connection between breast cancer and dental issues, the April 1997 *Townsend Letter* provides an anecdotal story. A female was diagnosed with breast cancer and while waiting for the tumor to be removed also discovered she had an abscessed tooth. After she had the dental procedure she had an X-ray taken as part of the pre-surgery routine. The X-ray showed a white streak from her tooth to the tumor. Puzzled by this strange X-ray her doctors delayed surgery. Four months later the tumor was gone. A later chapter addresses root canals, but suffice to say this story provides compelling evidence that there was a connection to a dental issue and one women's breast cancer.

LEUKEMIA

Leukemia is directly tied to mercury amalgams. Leukemia was first discovered in the early 1840's, a decade or so after the introduction of the mercury amalgam.

Dr. Pinto, a dentist, demonstrated the relationship in the early 1920's. He treated a six-year-old girl who had leukemia that complained her teeth hurt. Since he understood the relationship between mercury amalgams and disease, he removed her only mercury amalgam and she experienced spontaneous remission. Her doctors mocked the dental solution, so Dr. Pinto put a mercury amalgam back into her tooth and the leukemia returned. Successfully proving his theory, he removed the mercury amalgam, remission occurred again, and the child lived cancer free. This story has been repeated many times by other leukemia patients. However, all these anecdotal medical successes have never become part of any medical research.

Leukemia is typically diagnosed by using white blood cell count. The white blood cell count can either be very high or very low. This is a function of either an under active immune response or an over active response. The interesting relationship is that if normal white blood count is 5,000-6,000, pre and post amalgam response tends toward normalization. If a mercury toxic patient is low pre amalgam removal, it will migrate up post amalgam removal. And the vice versa also occurs. If white blood count is higher than the norm after removal it will reduce.

Other examples are well documented by Dr. Hal Huggins. A doctor with leukemia had his WBC drop from 176,000 to 59,000 after mercury amalgam removal. Another case showed a dramatic drop from 73,700 to 12,700. These stories suggest a relationship. White blood count is the primary indicator of leukemia, and white blood count, at least in small sample of leukemia patients, attempts to normalize after mercury amalgam removal. There are enough anecdotal stories to suggest a relationship between mercury amalgams and leukemia, at a minimum this relationship suggests that having mercury amalgams removed will improve your immune system. Of course, having a strong immune system is critical for recovery from any illness.

Leukemia is not only a childhood disease, but it is also certainly strikes young people at an alarming rate. If you think about it, it makes sense. Assume a responsible mother, with a number of mercury amalgams, passes mercury to the fetus, via the placenta during pregnancy. Then as a dedicated parent she nurses her child. We know this milk is contaminated with lots of mercury based on previously mentioned research. In fact, if mom has at least seven mercury amalgams her breast milk contains over 20 times more mercury than a nursing mom without mercury amalgams. And currently, 17% of all children between 2 and 4 years old have at least one amalgam filling and by the time a child is 8 years old, 52% have at least one mercury amalgam in their mouth. This is amazing since most manufacturers of amalgams contraindicate the use of mercury amalgams in children. Add to this the additional burden that mercury is contained in the plethora of vaccines that are administered, and this young innocent child has now been exposed to enough mercury to easily surpass any

135

government guideline. In fact there is enough mercury in this infant body to cause disease. The cause: mercury – the possible effect: leukemia, SIDS, A.D.D. or juvenile suicide and I am sure researchers can add to this list.

OTHER CANCERS

Most of the research between mercury and cancer has centered on breast cancer and leukemia. However, understanding the science of mercury and the human body, it is realistic to assume a relationship between mercury and stomach cancer, pancreatic cancer, liver cancer, and kidney cancer. These are all areas of the body that accumulate mercury.

Clearly, all cancer is not caused by mercury. But what if 1%, 10% or even 25% is caused by the initial release of mercury vapor from your dental fillings? There is enough evidence for the American Cancer Society or our government's primary research arm, The National Institute of Health, to spend a significant portion of its research money to investigate the relationship. How many lives could be saved and how much cancer could be prevented if the relationship was only 10%. If that 10% represented someone in your family, it would be the best research money ever spent.

Often times, it is easy to believe that everything causes cancer. Do not become disillusioned. Toxins create the opportunity for malignancy. However organic food, clean air and water, vitamins and minerals, love, fun, and laughter have never been associated with cancer. In many cases cancer is a choice based on life style. You can choose to make decisions that mitigate the risk of cancer and one of those is avoiding mercury amalgams.

AUTO IMMUNE DISEASES

When a person is diagnosed with M.S., ALS, Lupus, some forms of arthritis, epilepsy, diabetes, and Hashimoto's disease the common condition is that your immune system attacks seemingly healthy tissue. Somehow the markers on your tissue that normally keep this from occurring sends out a signal to your immune system that something is wrong, and an immune system attack commences. Not only is your immune system waging a war on sick and dying cells, which is its daily job, but it is also attacking seemingly healthy cells. It cannot differentiate; somehow purported cells are signaling for help from your immune system.

When this occurs various auto immune diseases are diagnosed. The major question is: why are cells in distress? One answer is maybe they are not "healthy" cells. Maybe your immune system is actually attacking compromised tissue. Mercury should be the focus of any explanation. We know that when mercury is released from your mercury amalgams it has a transport system to every cell. We also know it is a cytotoxin.

Traditional medicine believes that your immune system is getting false signals from cells and inappropriately attacks these healthy cells. However, maybe the cells are no longer healthy, once mercury attaches to the cell membrane the cell signals for help and a healthy immune system will attempt to "clean up" the changed cell. But how? We understand that finding a way to eliminate mercury is a huge challenge. Kidneys retain it, and the only potential avenue to exit is via the GI track. We also understand the kidney is an area where toxic buildup far exceeds the systems ability to eliminate it. As more mercury builds up throughout the body, mercury affects more cells and your immune system is now working overtime attacking seemingly healthy cells, albeit mercury-compromised, with reckless abandon. This is your immune system's job: to try and keep you healthy. When disease is finally diagnosed more and more functions are lost and finally death occurs. Traditional doctors blame an-out-of control immune system. I seriously doubt it. Your immune system is waging a war against something that will cause cell and tissue damage, and it is losing the battle.

M.S.

M.S. was described in 1818 in France and then in 1823 in England. It was first diagnosed in the mid 1830's. Again, it was discovered only a few years after the introduction of the dental amalgam. M.S. is an autoimmune disease that affects middle-age adults. M.S. affects females twice as much as males. It is the most common neurological disease in civilized countries. In less civilized countries the incidence of M.S. is often times non-existent. For example there are 12,000,000 Bantu's and no reported cases of M.S. Interestingly they have virtually no mercury amalgams. A couple of other facts make the previous comment interesting. One of the hallmarks of MS is that victims do not sweat, sweating is a great detoxifier, and the life expectancy after initial diagnosis is 21 years.

M.S. is a disease of the nervous system. The myelin sheaths that encircle the spinal cord and brain are compromised. Compromised or damaged by what is the critical question. In many documented cases the culprit was mercury. Multiple anecdotal stories assert that upon removal of dental amalgams wheelchair bound patients have walked out of the dental office.

The highest incidence of M.S. occurs in Northern Ireland and the Scottish Islands of Oakary and Shetland. Residents in these areas also have the most mercury amalgams per capita. Is this just an interesting relationship, or does it display a strong probability that the connection between M.S. and mercury is real?

A study was undertaken that compared blood chemistries and other criteria between M.S. patients with mercury amalgams and M.S. patients who had their amalgams removed. The M.S. patients with mercury amalgams had a lower red blood count, lower hemoglobin, lower hematocrit, lower T4, lower T lymphocytes, lower T8 suppressor cells, higher BUN, lower serum IgG, and higher levels of mercury in their hair analysis. In addition, this group had 33% more adverse health symptom flare-ups during the previous 12 months. In the M.S. group that had their mercury amalgams removed, 31% reported they felt better and 7% felt cured. No chelation or detoxification was used yet 38% felt better to some degree. This percent is far too large to suggest some type of placebo effect.

In another research study, it was discovered that M.S. patients have eight times more mercury in their cerebrospinal fluid than people without M.S. Remember the spinal cord is one of the affected areas referenced earlier.

In yet another study of 87 people with M.S., 83 had dental treatment with mercury just prior to the onset of M.S. Coincidence? I doubt it.

And, finally a dentist decided to replace 14 traditional mercury amalgams in a patient with the new high copper mercury amalgams. The unknowing patient was diagnosed with M.S. shortly thereafter. The individual discovered the relationship, had his fillings replaced with composites and detoxed with DMSA and DMPS. And guess what? His M.S. symptoms disappeared.

Research suggests essential fatty acids are important in relieving M.S. symptoms. Interestingly, this protocol is also important in mercury toxic patients!

The introduction of high copper amalgams magnified an already serious problem with the mercury amalgam. As mentioned previously in the mid 1970's a new mercury amalgam mix was introduced. It contained 30% copper and 50% mercury; significantly more copper than previous mixtures. In a study Brune demonstrated this mixture released 50 times more mercury than previous amalgams. In addition, it released a great deal of copper. We only need trace amounts of cooper – too much copper is toxic to the human body. These high copper amalgams are one of the reasons many mercury toxic patients are also copper toxic (and therefore zinc deficient). This may be one of the reasons M.S. is being diagnosed earlier and progressing more rapidly than in the past. To substantiate this study another study demonstrated elevated copper levels in M.S. victims.

Simply stated you cannot "catch" M.S. It develops based on a toxic exposure or exposures. The relationship to mercury from fish, vaccines, dental fillings or root canals demands investigation.

OTHER DISEASES

To the best of my knowledge there has been no direct research (a few articles suggesting a relationship) connecting Parkinson's, ALS, Colitis, and Crohns Disease to mercury. Epilepsy has one anecdotal story suggesting a person cured himself of epilepsy when he had his mercury amalgams removed. After the removal of his mercury amalgams, he has lived 15 years without a seizure, and he is in great health. There are stories of people with Lupus, which is considered incurable, regaining their health with mercury amalgam removal. Therefore it should not be considered incurable.

If I had research dollars, and each of these organizations have huge budgets, I would spend money determining if there was connection between mercury and the illness. The connection seems too obvious to ignore. Instead of spending millions of dollars searching for new drugs which suppress symptoms, the better solution is prevention.

HEART DISEASE ... A CLEAR CONNECTION

In the early 1900s no one experienced heart attacks, or at least heart disease was not a common cause of death. In fact, the first article regarding heart attacks was written in 1907. By the 1950s heart disease was a growing problem. Something had changed in our lives to create the massive growth in heart disease. In 1999 $300,000,000,000 was spent on 60,000,000 Americans with heart disease. As of today, 50% of all deaths are due to heart related disease. In less than 100 years heart disease has become the number one cause of death in the United States.

In order to determine why this happened, a massive study was undertaken, and it was determined that no one cause was the reason for the alarming increase in heart disease, but rather a number of risk factors accounted for the reasons for death by heart disease. These risk factors include elevated cholesterol, stress, smoking, obesity and the lack of exercise. Based on this study the American Heart Association is spending millions of dollars a year educating everyone on these new risks, risks that supposedly were not present early in the 20th century. And most of the world bought this study – hook, line and sinker.

In the early 1900's, when there was virtually no heart disease, the world diet consisted of a lot of fat. Every meal included meat of some type; breakfast was bacon and eggs. Average TSC was much higher than it is today. In fact there are tribes in Asia and Africa today whose diet is almost exclusively fat, yet these tribes experience no heart disease. The information regarding the dangers of smoking was non-existent – more people smoked. The exercise craze of the last 25 years was a distant thought to our grandparents. They did not run or bike everyday. And I believe The Great Depression created a lot more stress than today's economy. In spite of this, heart attacks did not exist a century ago. Nevertheless we labeled the growth of heart disease on these "new" risk factors. In reality these risk factors, if risk factors at all, were greater 100 years ago than today. This is not meant to dismiss that some of these risk factors may play a small part in heart disease, but to suggest that they account for the fact that 50% of the deaths this year will be because of these risk factors, is absurd. If so past generations should have had the same problems. These are not new risk factors. What is new since the early 1900's are all types of environmental pollution, toxins, processed, and mineral deficient foods. These seem to be better candidates for the higher incidence of heart disease than the types of food we eat.

In the early 1900's fewer people had dental work, thus they had fewer mercury amalgams. As the century progressed more mercury amalgams were placed, the fat controversy was born by the anti-fat proponents and heart disease escalated at an alarming rate. Is this interesting correlation or hypothetical crap?

A few studies may help answer the previous question.

o   Studies show that people with dental amalgams have higher blood pressure than control groups without amalgams.

o   A Russian scientist, Dr. Saytanov, exposed rabbits to mercury and he noted abnormal EKG's after exposure.

o   In 1984 Khayat and Dencker did studies with rats and monkeys and concluded the heart was a "target organ" of mercury.

o   In 1989 Yoshida exposed mother and baby guinea pigs to mercury vapor and found higher levels of mercury in the babies' heart and other organs than in their mothers.

o   A study demonstrated that mercury interferes with normal processing of nutrients that fuel the heart.

o   Washington University in St. Louis determined that mercury is found in the aorta and mercury also causes hypertension.

o   In 1989 Carmignani exposed rats to mercury in drinking water. The exposed rats had 20 times more mercury in heart tissue than the control group.

o   In 1989 Matsuo discovered mercury levels in the heart increase with age.

o   Mercury levels up to 22,000 times higher than normal were found in cardiac patients with ADCM.

o   In 1987 Freden put mercury amalgams in teeth of guinea pigs and sacrificed them at one, three, five, and ten days. Mercury accumulated rapidly in the heart tissue, even more than in the brain.

o   A Soviet Union study confirmed a number of earlier studies regarding mercury's effect on the cardiovascular system. Mercury had a number of negative effects:
    1.   Mercury increased blood pressure

141

      2. Mercury created abnormal EKG patterns

      3. Mercury damaged heart tissue.

o A different study exposed 665 subjects to mercury vapor. They exhibited the following changes: chest pain, heart palpitations, increased blood pressure, and irregular pulse.

o The Walter Reed Medical Center divided 48 animals into eight groups of six. They were placed in a circular plastic ring with a block of mercury amalgam in the center. The mercury amalgam was ground into small pieces, i.e., broken up, thus allowing mercury vapor to be released. Group one was not exposed to the mercury amalgam. Each group was sacrificed at time intervals after the grinding ceased. The group that was sacrificed immediately after the grinding stopped, thus had been exposed to mercury vapor for 30 minutes, and exhibited 81 times more mercury in the heart than the control group. In other words, mercury is easily absorbed and has a strong affinity for the heart muscle. Absorption in the heart was much greater than in the brain.

o Tests confirmed mercury attaches to SH sites in hemoglobin. Oxygen is lost, thus the reason for fatigue as a common symptom of mercury toxicity.

o Trekhtenberg discovered that mercury blocked nerve impulses from the Vagus Nerve to the heart tissue. Mercury interfered with the neurotransmitter, acetylcholine. Acetylcholine, an active protein site, is a SH protein, the interference with acetylcholine created a change in EKG, heart beat, and overall heart function diminished.

o Siberlud in 1990 studied blood pressure as it relates to mercury amalgams. There was significant increase in both systolic and diastolic blood pressure in volunteers with dental amalgams.

o Research conducted by The Nebraska Medical Foundation discovered young athletes that die suddenly from Osteopathic Dilated Cardiomyapathy have been shown to have 22000 times more mercury in their heart muscles than patients without cardiac conditions.

o In 2002, The Research Institute of Public Health at the University of Kuopio in Finland studied Finnish men and concluded that men with elevated mercury in their hair analysis had higher death rates from cardiovascular disease than men with low mercury in their hair analysis.

o In October 2002 the *Wall Street Journal* published research conducted from grants from the National Institute of Health. The bacteria associated with gum disease is linked to heart attack risk. Scientists at the Interscience Conference on Antimicrobial Agents presented evidence showing bacteria from periodontal disease promotes the build up of plaque which leads to heart attacks. Based on this information NIH is researching treatments such as tooth scaling, gum cleaning and antibiotics as ways to reduce the health risks this bacteria causes. No mention of the real cause – the mercury amalgam.

The above tests, studies and research prove mercury vapor causes heart problems. The marketing hype to lower cholesterol might actually be harming mercury toxic patients. Cholesterol might protect the body from mercury. Fat is critical for excretion of mercury. Have you ever known someone who went for a physical, discovered they had elevated cholesterol, went on a strict diet to lower cholesterol and died within 90 days of a heart attack? Or someone who could not reduce cholesterol with diet and took cholesterol lowering drug and subsequently died of a heart attack? I think we can all relate to the above scenarios.

Our ancestors had a much fatter diet then we do today. They had almost no incidence of heart disease. The escalation of heart disease occurred simultaneously with the growth of better dentistry, i.e., defined as saving more teeth, by using more mercury amalgams. More mercury amalgams equal more mercury vapor.

The suggestion that cholesterol actually protects our body from mercury should be investigated. Most cholesterol is made by our liver and not from the food we eat. If cholesterol is high, the liver has a role in that production, why is the liver producing excess cholesterol? If diet played such an important role in cholesterol why do vegetarians have high cholesterol?

I believe the American Heart Association needs to look at causes other than the risk factors they have identified. Managing these risk factors has not significantly changed the growth of heart disease. History provides a clue. What we need to determine is what happened between 1900 and 2000 to change our lives. Our diet did not deteriorate, smoking decreased, stress is hard to define, and exercise increased. One change is that our world has become much more toxic.

BLOOD SUGAR PROBLEMS; HYPOGLYCEMIA AND DIABETES

The liver regulates blood sugar. Hypoglycemia and diabetes are blood sugar issues and are opposite of each other. Some practitioners believe hypoglycemia is a precursor to diabetes and if hypoglycemia was universally recognized and tested the growth of diabetes would not only be drastically reduced, but type II situations might actually be eliminated. Currently 6% of Americans have diabetes, and that number is increasing every decade.

A glucose tolerance test determines blood sugar regulation. Low blood sugar creates hypoglycemia. A healthy liver can convert glycogen into glucose to bring blood sugar back to normal. When the liver is unable to do this blood sugar regulation is affected. The key element is the functioning of the liver. Remember the prime responsibility of the liver is detoxification and if the liver is compromised by an overburden of toxins, including mercury, then it cannot be healthy or efficient, and cannot convert glycogen to glucose. Thus the resulting blood sugar issues.

Some of the symptoms of hypoglycemia are confusion, persistent hunger, headaches, depression, irritability, temper, nervousness and fatigue. Interestingly, these are all common symptoms of mercury toxicity. Low blood sugar impacts the entire endocrine system.

Unlike its counterpart, diabetes, hypoglycemia is rather easy to remedy. First detoxify the liver. Second is a healthy diet. Eat some protein including whey and goat protein drinks. It is impossible too eat too many vegetables. Have one or two servings of fruit per day and eat only organic whole grains or sprouted whole grains. No refined carbohydrates, no fruit juices, no sugar, no alcohol, no additives and no caffeine. Initially it may be necessary to a small amount of protein and vegetables every couple of hours but within a few weeks you will see symptoms disappear or improve. The symptom that will disappear gradually but steadily is fatigue.

The timing of how often you need to eat is often a function of the glucose tolerance test. It is impossible to state a typical test result but lets assume during the four hour test the results of blood sugar mg/100 m is as follows, initial 86, 1 hour 140, 2nd hour 75, 3rd hour 60, 4th hour 75. The first hour is normal, a spike is expected and is normal in the first hour, and then the results should be about 100. In hour two the blood sugar falls and the liver is unable to correct the low levels. This means the person with these results probably needs to snack every two hours on some type of protein, for instance a few nuts etc. As your diet improves this two-hour period will extend. But, be vigilant and have some type of snack available based on your test results. The simple act of changing your diet will improve how your feel. As you change your diet concentrate on detoxifying your liver. The combination results in normal blood sugar levels.

Diabetes is the opposite of hypoglycemia. The hormone insulin regulates sugar metabolism. Insulin is released from the pancreas in response to a rise in blood sugar levels and attaches to receptor sites on cells. Diabetes happens when too little insulin is released. Diet is critical in controlling diabetes. Liver function remains important and insulin injections are typically necessary. Currently, 17 million Americans have diabetes, and that number is growing dramatically. The number of people with diabetes has tripled in the past 30 years and currently ranks as the most expensive health care problem in the United States. There are many anecdotal stories of people drastically reducing the amount of insulin they need when they eliminate mercury from their body. I have not heard or read of anyone curing diabetes with a detoxification program. Many practitioners believe juvenile diabetes is the direct result of vaccination programs, and if mercury were eliminated from vaccines, then the growth of this type of diabetes would be drastically reduced. The important aspect is to treat early blood sugar problems with a healthy diet and an aggressive liver detoxification program.

AUTISM

Autism has been referenced throughout the book. Autism did not exist 100 years ago. In fact autism did not exist prior to vaccines. Some parents testify that they have seen their child become autistic within days of receiving a vaccination. In the last 20 years there has been a 1000%

increase in autism. Changes in this two decade time period are a vast increase in vaccines containing thimersol, introduction of the MMR vaccine (studies have found the measles virus in the intestinal tract of children with autism – this is post MMR vaccination), multiple vaccines given at one time, an increase in breast feeding, and the increase in dentists filling baby teeth that have cavities with mercury amalgams.

One theory is that the dramatic rise in autism is based on the vast amount of environmental toxins a young person has to endure and a genetic make up that makes eliminating these toxins impossible.

An interesting anecdote: female dentists have the highest incidence of autistic children. No family or child should have to suffer the effects of autism. Simply put, drop the political crap, investigate thimersol, and mercury's impact on the neurological development of a child.

MYCOPLASMA AND VIRUSES

Mercury compromises every immune system. A compromised immune system provides an environment and opportunity for any pathogen to exist. Infections occur for a variety of reasons, but gastro intestinal dysbiosis and altered pH provide a terrain for opportunistic bacteria, viruses, fungi and infection to occur. Clearly number one on the list to remedy infection is to remove the toxin, i.e., the mercury amalgam, subsequently detoxify the body, and then allow a healthy immune system to combat the problems. Transfer factor as well as prescription drugs such as acyclovir will affect most viruses including most of the herpes strains and in some cases antibiotics are necessary to treat various bacteria. Simply put, a comprehensive blood test may very well indicate a variety of viruses and bacteria that have taken up residence in your body while mercury was compromising your immune system. It is necessary to eliminate them as quickly as possible.

In the last few years a variety of mycoplasma have been identified and some of these seem to proliferate after years of toxicity. Mycoplasma are the smallest self-replicating organism known in science. Not all mycoplasma are pathogenic but some create serious problems. The best known is the pneumonia mycoplasma that is pathogenic and identified with blood tests and treated rather easily with antibiotics. Others are equally as problematic, but much tougher to treat.

The mycoplasma organism has the capacity to invade cells, tissues, and blood thus producing systemic infections that effect most organs in the body. Mycoplasma steals vitamins, minerals, and amino acids from host cells. They are a parasitic bacteria, microscopic in size, and have rigid cell walls. They cause inflammation and release free radicals as well as suppress the immune system. They are pleomorphic (structurally changing) and thus they can easily avoid the immune system by hiding inside cell walls. In addition they can travel in platelets which have no immune response. This allows mycoplasma to travel undected through the circulation system. 75-85% of chronic fatigue, fibromyalgia, and chemical sensitivity victims test positive for a variety of mycoplasma, with fermentans the dominant strain. 90% of late stage cancer patients demonstrate mycoplasma infection, specifically fermentans. Also fermentans is the infection that most follows mercury toxicity. It requires a very elaborate blood test to identify this particular type of bacteria. IMMED, in Huntington Beach, CA, is a specialty laboratory that is an expert in mycoplasma research. Their web site is www.immed.org, and it provides a great deal of information.

Most of the autoimmune diseases have been associated with mycoplasma. In addition some of the symptoms of a mycoplasma infection are: joint pains, foot pain, thyroid problems, muscle aches, headaches, cognitive changes, fatigue, and gastro intestinal problems. One of the best indicators of mycoplasma problems, other than the blood test, is low and sometimes very low and natural killer cell function. A CBC can also provide insight. Elevated WBC, and elevated platelets are often indicative of infections. A long-term low-grade temperature is another sign of a mycoplasma infection.

In addition to the blood test to determine if bacterial infections exist it is also necessary to get a blood-clotting test from Hemex Laboratories in Phoenix, AZ. Mycoplasma will protect themselves from antibiotics, nutrients, and oxygen by triggering a clotting mechanism that acts as armor. The bacteria insulate themselves via this protective mechanism. This clotting mechanism produces soluble fibrin monomer, which are microscopic sheets that coat blood vessels. This reduces oxygen and nutrient exchange. The bacteria are now safe from protocols to destroy them. Hemex produces a test that will indicate if this condition exists. If it does exist it is necessary to eliminate the fibrin before antibiotics will work. Low doses of heparin will remove the protective shield and then protocols to eliminate the bacteria will succeed.

Some researchers believe there is a genetic relationship that creates the clotting mechanism. It appears those individuals with a European decent are most likely to fall victim to the following process; an infection activates the clotting described above, this creates the protective armor, restricts oxygen, and thus creates a myriad of symptoms including fatigue, muscle aches, low hormones, chemical sensitivities etc.

A doctor who uses dark field technology can save you a lot of money. From one drop of blood they can determine if this clotting mechanism exists, if so they know infection also exists. They can not determine the type of infection or the best antibiotic to treat it. But from one drop of blood from your finger they can predict with great certainly you have some type of infection.

Many people take antibiotics as the initial procedure to eradicate infections. It has to be done in concert with blood thinning medicines if the organism is going to be eliminated.

If a person is positive for pathogenic mycoplasms, elimination is a long tedious task. Mycoplasms are very difficult to destroy. Most protocols suggest at least six months, and possibly up to two years of antibiotic therapy. Typically, recent generations of antibiotics are effective in large amounts when used for extended periods of time. The course of antibiotics needs to be continuous with breaks only every 3-4 months. During the break periods determine what symptoms return. In a study when six-week cycles were used to evaluate the success of the antibiotic 100% of the study group relapsed after 6 weeks, 85% after 12 weeks, 27% after 30 weeks and 11% after 36 weeks. Thus it seems nine months of continuous usage helped 89% of the affected group. The most difficult to cure are the 11% and in those cases it might take up to 2 years of an antibiotic protocol. The antibiotics that are the most effective are: doxycycline, cipro, arithromycin, and zithromax. Dosages are high, and some practitioners continue to increase the dosage until severe symptoms disappear. Everyone will improve with the antibiotic, some more than others. But expect die off symptoms when high doses are used. The die-off symptoms decrease within a couple of weeks and slowly many symptoms show improvement. The most common die off symptoms are flu-like: fatigue, aches, chills and a fever. Also night sweats are very common. Hippocrates once stated; "Give me a chance to create a fever and I will cure any disease." The reaction to antibiotics demonstrates a couple of things; 1) an infection exists, 2) the antibiotics are working and 3) symptoms will slowly decrease. Do not fear the excess usage of antibiotics. It only helps and the fear that has been placed in our minds regarding the over usage of antibiotics is not relevant in this particular situation.

In addition to the antibiotics, it is critical to supplement large doses of probiotics. Antibiotics will negatively impact the benefical gut bacteria in your intestinal track. Simply replace the necessary probiotics. Mycoplasma is anaerobic so any type of oxygen therapy is very helpful. Most states regulate hyperbaric oxygen facilities although with a prescription, they are available to combat infection. Ozone therapy is also valuable and is available in many states. Hydrogen peroxide IV's, two hours plus, also have been reported to be helpful.

In the early 1900's HCL therapy was used to address bacterial infections and, with the advent of huge drug companies and the marketing of antibiotics, HCL therapy became obsolete. This occurred in spite of the great results and success HCL demonstrated over a 50 year time period. Finding a practitioner that uses HCL therapy either IV or IM would be a great compliment to the antibiotic and/or oxygen therapy you will need. Typically, diluted HCL is combined with procaine and injected into a muscle. HCL is a powerful antibiotic and can be very effective in combating mycoplasma.

Olive leaf extract's active ingredient is oleuropein. In 1960 research by UpJohn showed that oleuropein acid killed every virus tested. In the 1850's olive leaf was used to relieve fevers and malaria. Since then studies show it lowers blood pressure, increases blood flow in arteries, relieves irregular heart beats, and has strong antibacterial benefits. If you test positive for mycoplasma incorporate olive leaf extract into your protocol. The Bible has a great reference for olive leaf extract: "In the middle of its streets and on either side of the river has the tree of life, which bore 12 fruits, each tree yielding its fruit every month. The leaves of the tree were for the healing of the nations" (Revelations 22:2).

In addition to olive leaf extract add coconut oil to your daily protocol. The benefits of coconut oil are antimicrobal effects from the caprylic acid and lauric acid it contains. Coconut oil also enhances the immune system. Try and consume 4 tablespoons per day.

Finally there are clinics in Canada and Mexico that advertise a mycoplasma vaccine. The vaccine is mercury free (it is cultivated from your own blood) and is reported to stimulate the immune system against these micro organisms. In addition the vaccine causes a reduction in size of the organism, which allows for easier control and elimination. For more information search "mycoplasma vaccine."

Insulin Potentiated Theraphy (IPT) has been used for years as an alternative cancer treatment. It is now being used by IPT practitioners to address bacteria, viruses and fungus conditions. A small dose of insulin is given which creates a hypoglycemic condition. As your blood sugar drops, into the mid 30's, a variety of prescription drugs, herbs, and homepathics are administered IV and IM. Insulin increases cell permeability. When a cell is in this condition the effectiveness of any protocol increases. IPT offers a great option to those battling various infections without much success. I have heard of doctors who now administer DMPS while patients are in hypoglycemic state. This increases the elimination of mercury. When IPT is used to treat mycoplasma expect to have the same type of die symptoms described earlier.

If you have been sick for a while and already recognize that mercury was the cause, it would be worthwhile to rule out or address infections. You can supplement and detoxify for decades, but if infections are present it is necessary to eliminate them before you can reclaim your health.

Did you know that 4% of all hospital patients get an infection after they arrive at the hospital. This represents 2,000,000 Americans per year, 90,000 die from the infection. The solution; get out of the hospital as soon as you can.

Don't forget what it takes to get well.

.. DON'T BELIEVE TRADITIONAL MD'S REGARDING MERCURY. They are wrong.
.. DETOXIFYING FROM MERCURY IS A PROCESS, NOT AN EVENT. It takes time, in some cases years.
.. LEARN EVERYTHING YOU CAN FROM THIS BOOK AND OTHER SOURCES OF INFORMATION. Become an expert.
.. DON'T GIVE UP. Stay with the process of detoxification. You will see improvement eventually.

CHAPTER 11

*Who Is Wise And Understanding Among You? Let Him
Show It By His Good Life, By Deeds Done In The
Humility That Comes From Wisdom.*

ROOT CANALS – WORSE THAN AMALGAMS?

In the early 1900's research at the Mayo Clinic and research years later by Dr. Price and Dr. Meinig revealed that patients with root canals had more illness and disease than patients that had no root canals. The problem was not the root canal itself but bacteria that survived and mutated because of the root canal. Dr. Haley of the University of Kentucky has verified much of the earlier research in the late 1990's.

Dr. Price was employed at the National Dental Association Research Center in the 1920's and he performed fascinating and revealing research. He took a small portion of a root canalled tooth and inserted a fragment into a rabbit. Within a few weeks the rabbit had the same disease as the patient who had the root canalled tooth. This was repeated thousands of times so that science concluded that root canals, or rather the bacteria surrounding the root canal, cause serious disease. In Dr. Price's various publications, he describes over 100 diseases that were reversed once root canal teeth were extracted. These diseases include M.S., A.L.S., heart disease and various cancers.

The problem with root canals is that dead tissue remains in your mouth. The tooth is saved functionally, but the tooth and surrounding tissue is dead. This area becomes a breeding ground for highly toxic bacteria and toxins. It is estimated by the ADA that 30,000,000 root canals will be performed this year. Therefore 30,000,000 toxic teeth are releasing dangerous toxins. Remember, dentistry is big business and big business protects its territory at all costs. As an example, three years ago, Firestone created a massive cover-up to try and protect the fact that it produced and installed defective tires. The Attorney General is considering legal recourse. Dentistry is no better and no different.

The extensive research of the early 1900's should have eliminated root canals. Rather, we perpetuate and grow that business each year. Studies have provided more evidence of the dangers of root canals. First, five thousand root canal teeth were implanted in rabbits, all developed disease, the most common heart disease. A patient with kidney disease had a root canal tooth removed and subsequently the tooth was placed in 30 rabbits. All 30 rabbits died of kidney disease. This research was not random but convincing. In spite of 80 of years of research, we still place root canals in people's mouth, which leaves dead teeth in our mouth, which produce toxins that, in turn, produce disease.

Let's return to the dying tooth and the process of a root canal that creates the problem. A tooth is dying and thus causes pain. The death of the tooth can be due to an event, like a blow to the tooth or because of significant decay. In order to preserve the functionality of a tooth the dentist drills through the top of the tooth about 1/8 of an inch to the pulp chamber. Once the dentist has access to the nerve chamber, known as the pulp chamber, the dentist uses a small file to remove the contents of the chamber. At that point a valiant attempt is made to sterilize the area, but as you discover, it fails 100% of the time. The chamber is then filled with gutta percha. The gutta percha is heated and stuffed into the chamber.

The goal is to fill it so that it does not squirt out the bottom. To add insult to injury, mercury amalgam is typically used to fill the top portion of the tooth and a metal crown is added to the very top of the tooth. So we have gutta percha, mercury and a heavy metal crown of some type all residing in, or around a tooth.

The problem is that the gutta percha fills the pulp chamber, but has no access to the dentin tubules or the accessory canals of a tooth. These canals contain pulp material, but due to the microscopic size and impossible access, no filling material can be used on them. Thus, it is impossible to remove all the tissue in a tooth prior to filling it with gutta percha. This tissue becomes a site for bacteria and infection. How many canals does a tooth have that cannot be accessed by a dentist? Up to 75! Thus there are 75 potential sites per tooth for bacteria, toxins and infection. Additionally, after the gutta percha cools it shrinks in size and provides additional sites for bacteria.

Dr. Price researched the process of sterilization in root canals. He took 1,000 extracted teeth, sterilized them and then added the most caustic solutions available at that time (certainly nothing that could be used in a tooth that was in place in the mouth). 99% of the teeth tested positive for bacteria. He could not kill the bacteria. In a subsequent test, teeth were placed in autoclaves at extremely high temperatures. In this study no bacteria was discovered. Thus, bacteria in our root canal teeth can be eliminated, but not while the tooth still resides in our mouth.

The problem with bacteria that resides in dead tissue is that the bacteria are often anaerobic; they survive in the absence of oxygen. Anaerobic bacteria produce waste products far more toxic than traditional aerobic bacteria. Botulism is an example of anaerobic bacteria. This type of bacteria resides in multiple locations: in the tooth structure itself, the dentin tubules, the accessory canals and the periodontal ligament. A biopsy of the root canalled tooth demonstrates the toxic findings of anaerobic bacteria nearly 100% of the time. Most oral surgeons when they remove teeth do not remove the periodontal ligament. Failure to do so leaves a haven for bacteria, which cannot be accessed with traditional antibiotics.

Dr. Haley discovered that bacteria from root canalled teeth alter the functionality of many enzymes. Once an enzyme is compromised, the immune system is at risk and the potential for disease is real. It is obvious why so many spontaneous remissions of disease occur when root canalled teeth and periodontal ligaments are removed. The bacteria and the toxins that are produced are no longer compromising enzyme functionality. The opportunity for renewed health is now possible.

Dr. Meinig's *The Root Canal Coverup* suggests that 75% of the people's chronic and degenerative disease is caused by root canals. Let's assume his assumption is off by 50%, that's still an awful lot of disease that disappears if a root canal is either not performed or if the root canal tooth is extracted.

A study demonstrated that 90% of all cancer patients have root canals. This is compelling information since only about 25% of the population has root canals. This correlation is significant and should be viewed with a great deal of interest if you have a root canal or are considering one.

OK, root canals are dangerous, but what other options are available? The only answer is that the tooth and the periodontal ligament must be removed. Often times if the root canal has been in your mouth for a while the infection spreads to the jawbone and this area needs to be cleaned during the extraction process. This is often referred to as cavitation surgery for Neurologic Inducing Cavitation Osteomylitis (NICO).

Some alternative medical practitioners inject procaine into a root canal and wait and see if any of the patient's symptoms improve. If they do, it can be a sign of NICO. By removing the tooth and periodontal ligament, cleaning the entire socket (often times the bone is mush), and suturing the area, the symptoms are permanently resolved. An oral surgeon from your local yellow pages is not qualified to perform this surgery. All they do is numb the tooth and pull it. This requires expertise and to the best of my knowledge there are less than a dozen or so cavitation specialists in this country. Your mercury-free dentist should be able to refer you to one of them.

Now I have lost the tooth, what do I do to replace it? Dentures are the only option. Implants involve metals and they only cause new problems. There are some excellent dentures that are non-toxic, and although they do not have the same stability as a healthy tooth, they are safe and promote good health. As teeth are removed, it is imperative to reestablish the bite to its proper functioning or multiple problems can occur. Thus, do not ignore dentures or some type of partial once teeth are removed.

HOW MUCH DISCOMFORT WILL I EXPERIENCE DURING MY VARIOUS DENTAL WORK?

I have heard from so many patients that their biggest fear as it relates to mercury removal or cavitation surgery is the dentist. I can assure you your local mercury-free dentist that removes the mercury amalgam and the qualified oral surgeon who performs your cavitation surgery will make your fears disappear. Although you can experience periods of discomfort, your fears will prove unfounded. Qualified dentists have the medications and knowledge to almost guarantee you a pain-free experience and the light at the end of the tunnel is your health. GO FOR IT...

FLUORIDE – ANOTHER DENTAL TOXIN

The ADA has a great amount of research that substantiates the serious health consequences of mercury amalgams. They also ignore studies as it relates to root canals. Why then would the ADA be responsible when discussing fluoride?

Fluoride is a waste product of the aluminum and fertilizer industry. Prior to using it in drinking water, fluoride was sold as a poison for rats and insects. In fact, fluoride is considered more toxic than lead and about equal in toxicity to arsenic. The good news is that fluoride does a great job eliminating rats and other rodents. According to the Merck Manual fluoride is a lethal poison. Based on this background and the concern it should raise, did you know that 53% of Americans drink fluoridated water? Fluoridation occurs at the city, municipal and county water departments. *In Europe and Japan 98% of their population does not drink fluoridated water.* They have determined there are no benefits to fluoride in water and there are serious consequences when water is contaminated with fluoride.

The purported value of fluoride is that it reduces cavities in children. The reality is that fluoride does not reduce cavities, and in fact, may increase decay. Toronto has been fluoridating its water for 36 years; Vancouver has not been using fluoride. Toronto children have more cavities than children in Vancouver. Fluoride actually creates weaker teeth. Similar studies with 23000 elementary school children in Tucson, 22000 children in Japan, 400000 children in India and 25405 children in New Zealand substantiate the Canadian study. Fluoride increases decay when compared to fluoride free water.

The problem is not as simple as the fact that drinking water is compromised. Most commercial water is fluoridated. Fruit juice and soda also have fluoride contamination. Recently, a variety of soft drinks measured between 2.56 and 2.96 ppm of fluoride. Drinking water is supposed to be regulated at 1.0 ppm. Processed foods also measure positive for fluoride for the same reasons. Fluoride is also in some medications, such as Prozac, and in many household products. For instance, fluoride is in scotchguard and Teflon pans. Babies crawl on products treated with scotchguard. I cannot think of a person that needs fluoride less than a depressed person taking Prozac.

Fluoride, similar to mercury, is a slow poison. Studies suggest 50% of consumed fluoride remains in the human body. Consequences of fluoride usage include;
1. Fluorosis; (the damaging of the cells that form tooth enamel).
2. Five different studies document reduced I.Q. in children.
3. Elevated lead in children.

4. Reduced cellular functionality through enzyme inhibition.
5. Causes cancer.
6. Decreases bone strength by bone fluorosis.
7. Crosses the blood brain barrier becoming a neurotoxin and contributing to the entire spectrum of disease that affects the brain, including A.D.
8. Fluoride replaces iodine in the binding sites of the thyroid creating endocrine problems.

The FDA requires a warning label on all fluoride toothpastes. Basically it states that if a person swallows more than the amount used in brushing they should immediately call a Poison Control Center. This indicates a serious concern by the FDA. The message to an informed consumer is to avoid not only fluoride in toothpaste, but also in water, soft drinks, and any other form it is presented. It is a poison. Somehow, due only to politics, fluoride is used in many products, and only adds to the toxic burden our body has to deal with on a daily basis.

The only way to avoid cavities is through proper nutrition, and by balancing body chemistry. In addition flossing and brushing are critical in overall tooth health. Fluoride is no short cut; it actually produces additional decay since it interferes with proper body chemistry. The interesting issue regarding fluoridation is even advocates agree it only helps children under 12, yet cities and municipalities insist on making all ages drink water that has been poisoned.

Dr. John Yiannis compared cancer rates in the largest fluoridated and non-fluoridated cities in the United States. The cancer rates were similar prior to 1953, when fluoride was introduced. Cancer in fluoridated cities, however, outpaced cancer in non-fluoridated cities post 1953. A researcher at the National Cancer Institute concluded that fluoride causes more cancer deaths than any other toxin. He estimated 61,000 deaths in 1995.

In 1990 Dr. Marcus, a senior toxicologist at the EPA, discovered there was a cover up regarding fluoride usage. Studies proved fluoride caused cancer, birth defects and hip fractures. He exposed the EPA, was fired, and ultimately regained his job after filing a lawsuit. In spite of his research and the history of fluoride, it is clear politics will prevail over science. One half the population of the United States drinks the poison every day. There is nothing they can do about it. It is legislated by state

157

and local governments. Most filters are not capable of filtering fluoride from every day drinking water.

In order to combat the effects of fluoride take large amounts of Vitamin C and adequate amounts of magnesium. Most importantly, take iodine as a supplement. Iodine increases urinary excretion of fluoride. In addition, educate your city as to the dangers of fluoride, and avoid beverages made with fluoridated water. Finally, buy bottled water and distilled water whenever possible.

Last and most important, do not allow your dentist to give you any type of fluoride, which includes toothpaste, topical fluoride or brushing with a fluoride paste after a cleaning. Fluoride is poison - it should not be part of anyone's diet.

Another problem in 75% of the Unites States drinking water is chlorine. Chlorine has been used since 1908. Chlorine reacts with naturally occurring organic materials creating toxins that are carcinogenic. Ozone is a great disinfectant and should be substituted for chlorine whenever possible.

THE CONCEPT OF INFORMED CONSENT, OR IF YOU ARE GOING TO POISON US WE DESERVE TO KNOW HOW AND WHY.

Informed consent is a legal term, which means individuals **MUST** understand what medicals procedures are being offered, what options are available and what are the potential consequences of the various options. A medical doctor must explain the above and get a patient's permission prior to treatment.

Informed consent is a standard practice in medicine. The patient's approval is typically gained by the patient signing an informed consent form, or sometimes, if the procedure is not serious, the patient provides consent verbally. I suspect everyone remembers signing forms in a doctor's office prior to various tests being performed, in hospitals prior to X-rays being taken, and even nodding when a pharmacist provides us with possible side effects from a prescription. These are all types of informed consent. A person is being educated by an authority figure and is consenting to the action. Or in some cases they may choose not to go forward with the procedure based on the potential consequences. This is a choice.

Some additional types of informed consent are warnings on cigarette packages, NutraSweet labeling, non-prescription medicines, alcohol etc. Manufacturers that produce a product with potential harmful effects warn the public. In fact even products that are not deemed dangerous provide information to the public, so the public is informed. Go to any grocery store and every product lists the ingredients in their particular product. This is so the public can make informed decisions.

Less than 10% of American adults are aware that their dental amalgams contain mercury. The dental profession has effectively concealed this fact. This is in conflict with any definition of informed consent. A toxin represents 50% of the dental filling but this fact is cleverly concealed while poisoning everyone who has a single "silver filling."

Informed consent is non-existent in dental offices, except in California. Informed consent is non-existent in allergy offices where mercury is injected into patient's arms, and informed consent is rare in doctor's offices where babies are injected with thimersol as part of a rigorous mandatory vaccine program. City and county water departments do not warn you of the effects of fluoridation in their water supply. Why? If this is bother's you, and it should be, write the FDA or your local congressman.

California has taken a step toward resolving informed consent in their state. Prop 65 mandated California dentists post the following in their office: "This office uses amalgam filling materials which contain and expose you to a chemical known to cause birth defects and other reproductive harm. Please consult your dentist for more information." This is inadequate and misleading because it doesn't identify the "chemical" – the most toxic heavy metal, mercury.

But at least Prop 65 started the education process. No mention of mercury, just some chemical. Mercury is not a chemical but the measure provides some warning. The problem is that the warning appears aimed at pregnant or potentially pregnant women only. From the literature and science we know that the warning should be far more extensive.

The interesting aspect of the California legislation is that the California Dental Board never implemented the required informed consent. Most dental offices did not post the warning mandated by Prop 65. Thus in late 2001 the dental board was disbanded. A new board was installed and will have the mandate to post the warnings required by Prop 65. One of the new board members is a mercury free dentist. The new warning MUST read as follows, "Warning on dental amalgams, used in many dental fillings, causes exposure to mercury, a chemical known to the state of California to cause birth defects or other reproductive harm. Root canal treatments and restorations including fillings, crowns, and bridges, use chemicals known to the state of California to cause cancer. The US Food and Drug Administration has studied the situation and approved for use all dental restorative materials. Consult your dentist to determine which materials are appropriate for treatment."

Other states, due to consumer activism, are being forced to deal with the issue of mercury amalgams. Action is taking place in the following states: Washington, New Hampshire, Florida, Oregon, Maryland, Arizona, Maine, California and Iowa.

A grassroots organization, Consumers for Dental Choice, is beginning to file lawsuits in several states. Many of the legal actions are for violations of the Sherman Anti-Trust Act and violations of First Amendment rights.

The ADA uses its influence to get state run dental boards to adopt ADA guidelines thus restricting dentists from challenging the ADA position on mercury amalgams. When a dentist voices a concern regarding the use of mercury, his/her license to practice is challenged, and their reputation is smeared. Legal remedies are often costly for the dentist. Under gag orders disguised as "ethical rules," the dentist is not allowed to educate the patient, provide information, or research on the mercury amalgam. In addition, a dentist is not allowed to state that mercury vapor is released from every filling, and they are not allowed to advocate removal of mercury amalgams for health reasons. Dentists simply drill, fill (stuff mercury into the cavity) and bill the insurance company. In reality they are simply tooth mechanics. The preface to their name, "Doctor," should empower them to think, educate, and cure. But the ADA limits their power to simply fix a tooth by the standards they set.

In March 2002, Consumers for Dental Choice NW articulated legal arguments to the Attorney General in Oregon arguing for a rescission of gag orders in the State of Oregon. Under direction from the State Attorney General, the Oregon Dental Association rescinded the gag order. The argument from Consumers for Dental Choice NW was that the policy was an unconstitutional abridgment of free speech under both the state and federal constitutions. Oregon dentists may now speak freely about mercury amalgams, and the "M word" (mercury) can now be discussed with dental consumers. The hope is 49 other states follow Oregon's lead (Iowa is currently arguing a case similar to Oregon's argument and it appears their gag order will also become obsolete). The interesting aspect is that a dentist, prior to rescission, would not get into trouble with the local licensing board if he/she recommended mercury amalgam removal for cosmetic reasons! But if health reasons were discussed, it was a violation and a dentist's license could be revoked.

The dental profession should follow the medical practice in obtaining informed consent. Dentist should provide information to consumers so intelligent decisions can be made. The tobacco industry informs consumers their product is going to eventually kill some of them, but people still smoke. Mercury amalgams do the same thing. The dentist should provide the consumer with information regarding the mercury amalgam. Science and research will help consumers make an informed decision. That is not too much to ask for as consumers.

The ADA makes a huge amount of money when they provide a manufacturer with the "ADA approved" logo. Its power stretches beyond its ability to restrict dentist's First Amendment rights. The ADA controls research and accredits dental schools. The dangers of mercury amalgams are not part of any class at any dental school. The university teaches the ADA protocol. The ADA also controls dental products with the authority to restrict or issue an "ADA approved" logo on products. When an anti-amalgam dentist decides to challenge the ADA and the state licensing boards, the battle is truly analogous to David and Goliath. The issue at hand is the First Amendment. But state regulators control licenses and have the ability to make the fight a very expensive and risky one for a dentist.

As a consumer you should demand information. Every dentist's office should address the controversy, if it is still a controversy in your eyes, regarding mercury amalgams. The ADA can present its facts and opinions on mercury amalgams. Those that have grave concerns regarding mercury amalgams can present information regarding their position. But at a minimum, acceptable language that cannot be debated should be available and an informed consent form signed by every dental consumer.

An example of an acceptable informed consent agreement is as follows: "This dental office uses a filling material that is comprised of 50% mercury. Mercury is one of the most toxic heavy metal known to mankind. Research indicates mercury is released from your fillings over time and is absorbed into various organs. This office also has filling materials which do not contain mercury." If people chose to use mercury amalgams after this warning, so be it. Many people still smoke and most still consume too much sugar despite the dangers. Warnings are all that we can do as responsible watchdogs.

The ADA is speaking out of both sides of its mouth. The interesting aspect of the ADA position is that they support mercury amalgam usage but they assume no responsibility when litigation occurs. A few years ago the ADA, in defending itself in a mercury amalgam poisoning case, asserted that it "... owes no duty of care to protect the public from allegedly dangerous products used by dentists because the ADA did not manufacturer, design, supply or install the mercury containing amalgam ... (and) does not control those who do." Interpreting this statement: the ADA researches products, endorses a product, demands its usage by dentists, penalizes dentists who don't use it, but has no duty to warn consumers of alleged dangers of any of the products. To summarize, every mercury amalgam dentist will be on his/her own when lawsuits proliferate. A dentist should not expect protection from the ADA.

For years the tobacco industry fought against warning labels on cigarettes. The reason was simple. Maybe not morally or ethically appropriate but nevertheless they opposed warning labels. If they made the public aware of the dangers of their product, smoking would decrease. Eventually consumers were made aware, in writing, on all packages of cigarettes about risks of tobacco smoke. The price people paid for this delay or admission of the health risk of smoking was in many cases with their life. Today the ADA is fighting informed consent. The reason is familiar: money. Denying the research and delaying the inevitable will cost many their quality of life and in many cases cause illness, disease and death.

Success depends on commitments to the four principals discussed through out this book:

.. DON'T BELIEVE TRADITIONAL MD'S REGARDING MERCURY. They are wrong.
.. DETOXIFYING FROM MERCURY IS A PROCESS, NOT AN EVENT. It takes time, in some years.
.. LEARN EVRYTHING YOU CAN FROM THIS BOOK AND OTHER SOURCES OF INFORMATION. Become an expert.
.. DON'T GIVE UP. Stay with the process of detoxification. You will see improvement eventually.

CHAPTER 12

If Any Of You Lacks Wisdom, He Should Ask God, Who Gives Generously To All Without Finding Fault, And It Will Be Given To Him

WHAT ELSE DO I NEED TO KNOW?

You should keep a journal or a notebook that lists symptoms, and make notes of improvements. This will be important as you progress through your journey of healing. If you get frustrated, read the journal from the beginning. Seeing success helps you stay on the track toward full health.

Almost everyone that is mercury toxic is lead toxic. The first thing to do is concentrate on getting the mercury out of your system. Again DMPS or DMSA is the best chelator for this purpose. A chelator that is often used for lead removal is EDTA. Never use EDTA until the mercury is removed. While you are detoxifying, avoid all products that might contain lead. One of the major sources of lead is commercial hair dyes. If you use a hair dye visit your local health food store and find one that is non-toxic. Also DMSA is an excellent chelator of lead.

Fasting is a popular detoxification protocol. If healthy, simply performing a fasting in order to add zest and vitality to your life is probably a good idea. However, if you are moderately to severely toxic it is probably a bad idea. Not eating can cause a strain on detoxification organs and if there are blood sugar problems (and there usually are) maintaining a constant blood sugar is a necessity. Fasting will interfere with mercury chelation.

Some people have tried essential oils and claim they are excellent chelators. At this point, there is very limited research to support the claim, but it might be worth pursuing. Some initial research suggests essential oils can not only help detoxification but also eliminate bacteria. Essential oils are very small molecules thus they are easily absorbed. In 30 minutes every cell is affected. Topically or orally they work equally as well since essential oils will move into the body thorough the skin rapidly.

Avoid toxic substances in household cleaners and especially new carpeting. Never let a baby crawl on new carpeting. The toxins in carpeting create serious problems for the mercury toxic individual, and infants are exposed to a plethora of toxins.

Exercise is important. Do not enter into a strenuous program but a daily walk, yoga, biking, swimming (not in a chlorinated pool) or a stretching program all have value.

In addition to lead problems, many people also have aluminum toxicity. Aluminum problems have been associated with Alzheimer's disease and thus avoid aluminum cookware and antacids. If you have excessive aluminum in your hair analysis, be sure to take magnesium and add malic acid. Malic acid is an excellent chelator of aluminum and dosages vary between 800-2400 mgs per day. The amino acid glycine is also an excellent chelator of aluminum. Take 2-3 grams twice a day. However in order to eliminate any metal your liver must be functioning appropriately.

Chelators attract heavy metals in a particular order. Thus as you progress through various DMPS and DMSA procedures you will note different amounts of heavy metals that are eliminated from your system. The order you should expect, from the beginning to end:
> Mercury
> Copper
> Lead
> Cadmium
> Tin
> Aluminum

Think of this in terms of a bucket. Every DMPS/DMSA procedure empties some of the toxins in the bucket. At the top of the bucket is mercury and initially mercury is the primary target of the chelators, although you will find some lead coming out early. Subsequently, DMPS and DMSA empty the bucket as described above. The challenge for each patient is to determine how long it will take for the chelators to empty your toxic bucket. The good news is that many books describe patients that get well very quickly. The bad news is that for most of us we can expect years before we eliminate all the toxins in our body. And health cannot be restored until the toxins are removed.

Once the mercury is removed you may still have symptoms. The reason for this is that other heavy metals have accumulated in your system. Once mercury compromised your immune system, other heavy metals that normally would have been released have been stored in your body. In addition symptoms created by bacteria infections can mimic mercury symptoms. The following chelators are effective in removing other toxic metals.

Aluminum: DMSA, penacillamine, malic acid, glycine
Copper: DMPS, DMSA, additional zinc, carnosine
Lead: DMSA, EDTA, Vitamin C
Cadmium: DMPS, DMSA, Vitamin C
Tin: DMPS, DMSA
Iron: EDTA

Is it possible that high cholesterol is associated with mercury? In my case, my cholesterol gradually fell from 350 to 211 when my mercury amalgams were removed. No change in diet. Interestingly recent studies that were suppose to support the relationship between fat and cholesterol failed to prove that theory. The famous Framingham Study started in 1948 compared people who had high cholesterol diets with those that had low cholesterol diets. Those on the high cholesterol diet had lower cholesterol levels. And the "French Paradox": why do the French who eat a diet high in cholesterol have lower levels of cholesterol than most?

In some studies vegetarians have shown high cholesterol levels and maybe the most important study linked high cholesterol levels with an imbalance in body chemistries. And heavy metal toxicity is one of the primary causes of vitamin and mineral imbalances. In many cases cholesterol is variable depending on detoxification issues. For instance, if you are releasing huge amounts of metals, cholesterol may spike to a high number then return to normal when the detoxification protocol is over. The speculation is that cholesterol is acting in the role as an antioxidant during the period of aggressive detoxification, or at times when disease, bacteria or viruses are present. The reality is that most cholesterol is made in the liver and is not a function of diet.

Continuing a theoretical discussion of cholesterol; oat bran and other fibers have been shown to decrease cholesterol when taken regularly. Is it possible that the fiber effects of oat bran actually remove toxins from your intestinal tract thus lowering cholesterol? As stated earlier, a diet high in fiber is critical for all toxic individuals. Large regular bowel movements are necessary to remove toxins. Oat bran is a great fiber that helps increase the frequency of bowel movements. Is it possible researchers missed this key variable in the study of fiber's impact on cholesterol? As a final note, when you increase your fiber intake be sure to drink 6-10 glasses of filtered water per day.

As mentioned earlier fish is a source of mercury. While you are detoxifying do not eat fish. Why burden your body with trying to remove additional mercury when it cannot even release the amount you currently have stored in your body?

The following table represents daily mercury retention:

	Mercury Retention
dental amalgams	3.0-17.0
fish	2.3
other food	0.25
water	0.0035
air	0.001

Based on this table I think it is fair to suggest that if you avoid mercury amalgams, do not eat fish and drink filtered water, in conjunction with DMPS and DMSA then you eliminate more mercury than you ingest.

Eat smart; your diet should include some protein, lots of vegetables, and a small amount of fruit. Do not consume sugar, alcohol, and definitely stop smoking if you are a smoker.

Avoid tap water. Drink either distilled water or filtered water. Tap water is filled with a variety of heavy metals. Don't increase the burden on your system. But drink lots of good water; as much as you can every day. Multi-Pure introduced a system designed to eliminate mercury from your tap water. In addition it eliminates numerous other heavy metals and bacteria.

It is important that your lymph system is working properly. There are a number of good books on your lymph system but some of the better things to do are walking, deep breathing, exercising on a re-bounder, massage, accupressure, and Trager therapy. Each of these will stimulate your lymph system and thus be another channel to remove mercury from your body. If you schedule a massage prior to your colonic you will improve lymphatic drainage. When this occurs you should start noticing significant improvements in your health.

Use castor oil packs as frequently as possible; 60-90 minutes before bed soak a wool cloth in castor oil, place it on your abdomen with coverage over your liver and abdomen. Place a towel over the wool, then place a heating pad (on high if possible) over the towel. This is a great protocol and will provide outstanding results. Many liver cleansing programs recommend castor oil packs for 7-10 days prior to the actual cleanse.

If you are chemically sensitive liver detoxification is critical. Support your liver with milk thistle, increase zinc and magnesium if they are low in your hair analysis, and use an infrared sauna as often as possible. In addition, be sure you are getting as many of the sulfur based amino acids as possible, particularly taurine. Investigate mycoplasma infections. And finally, do liver cleanses and colonics. Chemical sensitivities make life miserable. It is possible to overcome them with aggressive liver detoxification.

Some people suffer from galvanic reaction. This occurs when two or more metals combine with saliva to create a battery effect in your mouth. Amalgams have at least two metals in them; this painful symptom is a function of multiple metals in the mouth and is eliminated when mercury amalgams are removed.

If a person needs braces, find a dentist who uses metal free products. Braces contain nickel, which is a carcinogen, and should be avoided.

Many dentists' coat children's teeth with a compound called bisphenol-A in order prevent cavities. Studies from both Spain and Tufts University found this substance to be an estogenic mimic that could cause cancer. Similar to other dental research the ADA has chosen to ignore this information and defends the practice of applying a potential cancer causing coating to children's teeth.

OK, I'M GETTING THERE...WHAT ARE THE MOST COMMONLY ASKED QUESTIONS?

How much mercury is too much?

The answer is simple. The goal should be zero parts per billion. U.S. regulators can not agree on acceptable levels – various agencies have ranges from 25-50 ppb. Germany has standard of 10 ppb and Switzerland has a uniform standard of 1 ppb. The real question is why the U.S. has a standard 50 times greater than Switzerland. Is "U.S. mercury" less toxic than "Swiss mercury"? The half life of mercury is 87 years regardless of where you live.

Why does mercury replace healthy minerals in cells and tissues?

First, mercury has access to every cell, tissue and organ in the body. Second, mercury is an element and found in the periodic table just like, copper, zinc, and manganese. As a heavy metal, it replaces healthy, required minerals. In this case mercury is available and thus it replaces the healthy mineral. In many cases it is zinc or magnesium, which is replaced with mercury. When this substitution takes place it disrupts enzymes, hormones, and all the metabolic processes in the human body.

What side effects can I expect from DMPS?

For the most part the side effects are minimal to non-existent, providing caution is used and you start with small doses and ramp up very gradually. DMPS has been used extensively in Europe for many years. You can expect fatigue and potentially some restless sleep the night of your injections. Some people also develop a mercury rash. This is good news disguised as an itch. The mercury has been mobilized by the DMPS and your body is trying to eliminate the toxin. During this process some people get a bright red rash that is very itchy and can cover a large part of the body. You also may experience your blood pressure lowering and your pulse increasing. Another side effect common with oral DMPS is canker sores. If you plan to take oral DMPS take it in conjunction with the amino acid lysine. As your intestinal flora changes, and balances, canker sores are often times a byproduct. Lysine works better than any prescription medication available to help with the discomfort of canker sores.

How do I improve my oxyhemoglobin saturation?

One of the tests to determine mercury toxicity is the oxyhemoglobin test/venous blood gas mentioned earlier in the book. You should see improvement in this number as you migrate through detoxification. However, sometimes you will find yourself on a roller coaster, i.e., the number moving up and down. This can be discouraging and the reason for this is that it's critical to use any chelator frequently in order to move the mercury out of your body. If you mobilize the mercury but its does not chelate out, then the mercury simply finds a new home in your body. Do not stop various forms of chelation until you get your oxyhemoglobin to at least 70% and it stays there for 3 months, your hair analysis shows no heavy metals at toxic levels and you are symptom free.

How else can I eliminate mercury from my body?

Large amounts of vitamin C help, particularly with DMPS or DMSA. This assumes that you do not have a severe pH problem. Lots of fiber including psylium shortens transit time in your bowels and this is also very helpful. Many people suffer from constipation and diarrhea, and psylium helps reeducate your bowels and creates frequent and predictable bowel movements while eliminating toxins. Some people alternate between diarrhea and constipation during their detoxification process. This is simply part of the process. If you find that you are in a prolonged period of constipation do not take a fiber supplement and follow the instructions of your colon hydro therapist. It is important to keep your bowels moving. The reasons for this are multiple, but from a mercury perspective once you find a way to extract it from your tissue and cells you need to eliminate it from your body before it is reabsorbed. As mentioned previously, German research has stated that it may take up to 300 colonics before your intestines can start functioning properly. Some practitioners also advise sweat therapy. Just make sure that you add back all the good minerals that you sweat out. These include magnesium, calcium and zinc. Remember there are only three ways to eliminate a toxin from your body: kidneys, bowels and skin. Try each of them.

Additionally it's worth experimenting with acupuncture and massage. Both have proponents that suggest they help eliminate heavy metals from your body. Also try a detoxifying bath using Epson salts, hydrogen peroxide, apple cider vinegar, and baking soda. Be sure the baking soda is aluminum free, some report this bath to be an excellent chelator. A note on Epsom salts; some liver cleanses use Epsom salts orally, never do this. It can be very toxic to the gastro intestinal system. Substitute magnesium citrate.

Some people seem allergic to vitamins and minerals when they start the detox process. What can be done to solve this problem?

I do not think anyone is allergic to vitamins and minerals. Think about it for a minute. Do you think we were really designed to be allergic to vitamin C? Now we might be allergic to vitamin C that is derived from corn but it is highly unlikely someone is reacting to vitamins and minerals. I think there is a better chance that by supplementing valuable nutrition into your toxic body your body is simply reacting. It makes sense. When your body was exposed to mercury it reacted. It made you sick. Now that you are changing the pattern your body is reacting to the good stuff. My suggestion is to reduce the amount of vitamins and let your body adjust slowly.

What diseases have been associated with mercury toxicity?

Research has linked the following disorders/diseases with mercury.
- Alzheimer's
- M.S.
- Parkinson's
- Lou Gehrig's Disease
- Cancer
- Heart Attacks

This is frightening. Each of the above has some type of research that draws a relationship between the disease and mercury. Why doesn't anyone take the limited research that has been done and expand the analysis? Baffling, but not really that surprising.

Most research money comes from the government and pharmaceutical companies. This kind of research results in a new drug, which addresses symptoms, not cures, and generates billions of dollars of income to pharmaceutical companies.

My dentist is having a problem getting me numb prior to doing his dental work?

This is probably low magnesium. Low levels of magnesium causes nerves to become supersensitive to pain. The other possibility is an underlying infection; you have either a root canal or a deep mercury amalgam that is killing the tooth and causing an infection. Make an appointment with an alternative oral surgeon and determine if cavitation surgery is necessary. It is also possible that excess copper is the problem. Elevated copper decreases a person's pain tolerance. What is uncomfortable for a person with normal body chemistry is agonizingly painful with someone with elevated copper. Also low levels of B12 can cause the problem. But I'd start with low magnesium levels as the reason.

Is there a relationship between mercury toxicity and candida?

The easy answer is yes. Remember mercury compromises your immune system and makes your body a host for all kinds of bad things. This could include parasites as well as yeast overgrowth. Your internal ecosystem has been changed and now you have an environment where yeast can multiply. If you have been treated for candida and had only limited success it's a good bet that candida is only a symptom. The cause might be mercury.

Various mycoplasma bacteria that are present in the gastric system are another potential cause of candida. It's wise to test for these organisms as part of your overall analysis to determine if mycoplasma is part of the problem. In addition, candida often exists simply because of diet, the over usage of antibiotics or stress. And finally, if mercury has accumulated in your tissues it's a fair guess that you will need to chelate the mercury out of your body before you can address candida. If you are mercury toxic there is a good chance you also have yeast overgrowth. It is also a good bet that you will not get the yeast under control under you eliminate the mercury. Then you can attack the yeast with all the traditional yeast protocols.

Typical symptoms of candida are craving for sugar and products that contain yeast (bread, beer etc), depression, anxiety, insomnia, and hormonal problems. There are also numerous other symptoms that are associated with candida. Typically alcohol, sugar and bread products will magnify symptoms related to candida thus it's best to avoid these products while you rid yourself of this toxin. (I believe yeast overgrowth is a toxin just like heavy metals. This overgrowth creates an imbalance; your internal ecosystem is out of balance and normal health is impossible.) Recent information suggests that yeast overgrowth is a result of too many antibiotics, birth control pills, medicines, and heavy metals that affect the proper balance in your intestinal tract. Once yeast is allowed to multiply it affects many functions since the yeast itself output a toxin that is carried in your bloodstream.

Unfortunately, mainstream medicine does not believe that candida exists. But it does and many people could be much healthier if they tried protocols to eliminate the excess yeast. Typically a person can see results in a few weeks and dramatic changes in only a few months. What a travesty that doctors don't suggest patients at least try this remedy. I recently read an article that suggested over 50% of the people that are taking Prozac are doing so because of either mercury poisoning or candida. And the author suggested the percentage might be low. In other words, depression is simply a symptom. The cause is mercury and/or candida or both. Also, most studies suggest that females are at a greater risk for candida than men. This may have to do with the negative impact of birth control pills. Similar to mercury toxicity, Candida is a slow process. Initially the problems or symptoms can be overlooked but over time symptoms increase and eventually can be debilitating. Its a travesty so many people have lost their quality of life when a simple diet change and some anti fungal medicine would allow them to be reborn. I wonder how much the stock value of Lily (Lily is the drug manufacturer of Prozac) would tumble if this fact was substantiated? If you suspect Candida might be your problem please buy one of Dr. Crook's books, either the *Yeast Connection* or the *Yeast Connection and Women.*

What's the relationship between fibromyalgia and mercury?

Fibromyalgia is chronic muscle pain accompanied by fatigue that has no obvious cause and has no cure according to the AMA. It typically affects the back, neck and shoulders. This discomfort is often described as a stabbing feeling, throbbing or stiffness. Often times many other symptoms exist in conjunction with fibromyalgia. Interestingly, all the symptoms are the same symptoms that exist with mercury and aluminum toxicity. It is not surprising that a number of practitioners correlate fibromyalgia with mercury toxicity or other heavy metals. In fact, there is a reason to do so. Most suffers of fibromyalgia have a sodium/potassium imbalance, high calcium and high copper in their hair analysis. These are also typical imbalances in mercury toxicity.

I know of at least three people who have overcome fibromyalgia with DMPS/DMSA treatments. It would appear in some people that fibromyalgia is one of the latter symptoms of mercury toxicity. In other words, many symptoms precede this symptom and somehow mercury has found its way deeper into our cellular tissue. Unlike the mainstream doctor who simply tells that the only solution is to live with it, I believe symptoms can be relieved and ultimately eliminated by using protocols suggested in this book. Also, consider Shiatsu massage. This stimulates muscles and this stimulation helps release stored toxins.

Do I need to avoid industrial chemicals?

If you are toxic, albeit with mercury, other metals or chemicals it severely impairs your ability to absorb nutrients. Detoxification is a wonderful double edge sword; you eliminate toxic disease producing materials and create the opportunity for energy producing vitamins and minerals to take their place. Any type of industrial chemical will hinder this process.

Approximately 70,000 toxic chemicals are used in commerce today. Producing poisons is big business. Combating their affects on us is a big responsibility. For instance, paint contains a variety of toxic chemicals and 90 percent of Americans have measurable amounts of paint toxins in their bodies. There are a number of toxic free paints available and everyone should be using them in spite of the cost difference and limited color varieties available.

Farmers spend over $25,000,000,000 on pesticides. However, less than 0.1% reaches the targeted bugs. The money spent is inefficient, but remember the pesticide is a toxin and is toxic to everyone who is exposed to it. If this does not convince you to eat organic then nothing will convince you.

Chemicals only add to the toxic burden mercury creates. Avoid every chemical, pesticide and poison as much as possible.

Through DMPS/DMSA and other detoxification efforts I no longer show mercury in my challenge but I still have symptoms?

Remember DMPS is an excellent chelator of mercury but does a poor job on other heavy metals. If your hair analysis shows you still have aluminum, lead, copper switch to other chelating agents as a way to eliminate these heavy metals. And always use colonic therapy while chelating

How do I pay for mercury detoxification? This does not sound cheap?

The answer to the latter is that it is expensive. The dental portion of your procedure is only part one. The biggest expense is getting your body healed. DMPS is expensive, the vitamin IV's are not cheap, and the amount and quantities of supplements become costly. The best starting point is to go to your insurance company and show them your history, all previous procedures etc, as well as test or tests that indicate mercury might be the problem. Maybe just maybe, you will receive cooperation. Depending on the age of the amalgams your insurance might pay for replacements,, your insurance should cover some lab tests.

The next step is to go forth with the mercury detoxification, and try to convince your doctor or clinic to work with you on a payment plan. Then as you start feeling better get certain tests repeated that hopefully show improvement and take these tests to your insurance company and hope for better luck this time with tangible tests results. If your insurance company is still uncooperative then you can always think about litigation. This is sensitive since you will be suing the insurance company of your employer; think this through, the political implications are obvious.

A great solution is to sue the ADA, your dentist, the AMA, and anyone else you can think of. They have harmed you and caused disease and illness. Tobacco companies have paid, and I guarantee Firestone will have significant pay-outs based on the failure of their tires. The act of putting a poison in your mouth and seems more dangerous than either of the latter. Clearly this option takes a great deal of time, money and recourses. But hopefully someone will be angry enough and have the time, money and resources to pursue this option.

The other options are to get a second mortgage on your home if necessary to pay for this expense, or ask for help from family members. Hopefully you have saved for a rainy day and I can assure you this qualifies as a rainy day.

How long will it take to get well?

I wish I could answer this question. I cannot and no one can. Some people never get better. Others improve somewhat and others given time recover fully. I can say this, if you are young you will recover more quickly than if you are older. The fewer mercury fillings the better, you will recover more quickly with less mercury vapor releasing everyday. The more fillings the more protracted the recovery period. What kind of physical condition were you in before the symptoms started appearing? If you exercised, ate intelligently, etc. you are better prepared for a faster recovery. Additionally how long did it take to diagnose mercury as the cause? The longer you continued to inhale toxins and store them in your cells the longer it takes to dig them out. It's a fact that chewing releases large amounts of mercury. And we all ate three meals a day for how many years after we had our mercury amalgams? Also did you chew gum ... if you did that caused mercury to be released faster. If you still do stop now. My initial DMPS challenge measured 264 parts per billion of mercury and 528 mcg of mercury in 24 hours. These are astronomical numbers and no doctor I've seen has seen higher numbers. A number of doctors told me I should be dead. It took about 24 months of DMPS and other detoxification procedures discussed in this book before I started seeing relief. And it took another five years before my symptoms were manageable. If it worked for me with the levels of mercury I had it will work for you. Be patient, and it will be worth the effort.

What role does heredity play in mercury toxicity?

I believe that it is critical. If you are mercury toxic I bet you can take a look at your family history and determine who might have been affected by mercury. Hopefully these members of your family are still alive and can take at advantage of your knowledge. Unfortunately, I also bet there are deceased members of your family that you can ponder if mercury toxicity was a precursor to their death. The message is help those that you can and that are open minded enough to listen to you. Never put mercury amalgams in your children's mouth. As mentioned earlier in the book, certain recently identified genes create the problem of restricting the release of mercury naturally. Thus, the potential reason that one person can have a mouthful of mercury amalgams with seemingly no health problems while others have a few mercury amalgams and have a plethora of symptoms.

When will the AMA and the ADA recognize the health problems caused by mercury?

Who knows? Everyday that goes by just increases the magnitude of malpractice that they are committing. When the health effects of mercury amalgams are proven the public outrage will be headline news for months. Just think about the crisis the tobacco industry is involved in based on the fact that they knew they were selling an addictive product that is a carcinogen. Tobacco companies are settling with state and federal entities for millions of dollars. When consumers realize the AMA and the ADA knew about the hazards of mercury amalgams and allowed dentists to knowingly poison the population they were suppose to protect, the settlements the tobacco companies reached will seem like pocket change.

Currently Californian Congresswoman Diane Watson and Indiana Congressman Dan Burton have introduced a federal bill to ban mercury amalgams in the United States. In spite of their heroic attempts to change things my bet is that politics and the position of authority that the ADA enjoys will prevail. Nevertheless awareness is being raised by on this bill.

What can I do to help?

If you are in the midst of mercury detoxification this may not mean much to you. Use your energy to get well. I guarantee after you regain your health you will want to do something. Write to anyone and everyone – your congressman, your senators, the Surgeon General, the National Institute of Health, the American Cancer Society, the AMA, the ADA and every doctor that unsuccessfully treated you. Who knows, you just might get one or two of them to listen to you. Talk to anyone that will listen. Get the message out. Finally if you ever are in the financial position to help a mercury toxic person who does not have the financial means to pay for the procedures help them out.

Any final thoughts?

Just one – pray. Pray for yourself, pray for others. This is a powerful tool. It's been interesting to me as I have migrated through the challenges of getting heavy metals out of my system how many Christians I have met.

These are people who have been told to give up by the traditional medical profession, who have been told they are nuts, who have been told to live their life as best they can since no one can help them, and who have suffered monumental personal setbacks. Yet for some reason these same people have somehow gotten well, they never gave up and each has a pray routine. There is research to back up this bit of advice - try it. It cannot hurt and it may give you the strength to win this battle. Who knows maybe the person listening to these prayers is an advocate of mercury free dentistry? No father wants his children to suffer from an illness that is totally preventable. And I don't believe our Father does either.

GOOD LUCK ON YOUR JOURNEY TO BETTER HEALTH

Godspeed to everyone who is on this arduous journey to better health. I sincerely hope this book has provided some insight to each reader. If it helps just one person regain their health it was worth the effort. I plan to update this periodically and I would appreciate it if everyone who has knowledge, thoughts, or ideas to forward them to me so we can evaluate them and include them in future editions. Quite frankly, until mainstream medicine is prepared to assist us we need to educate ourselves.

CONCLUSION: FIRST DO NO HARM

As discussed earlier the mixture of mercury and any other metal or metals is an amalgam. Amalgam usage in the United States started in 1833. Since that time the usage of mercury amalgams has caused widespread controversy with 100% of the research supporting the fact that mercury in the dental mixture "leaks" and causes disease and illness. The policing agencies responsible for establishing the toxicity of this material are the ADA and NIDR. The ADA has never funded research to prove the safety of mercury amalgams. The mercury amalgam has been used for over 170 years in this country. NIDR has recently funded a study, which proved mercury vapor is released from amalgams. Their mission is dental material compatibility. Since their research no policy statement has been issued.

The ADA is a trade organization, and it claims it does not dictate policy. The ADA is a strange and complex organization. The ADA harasses dentists for not using mercury amalgams. The ADA has been instrumental in dentists losing their license to practice simply because a dentist believes mercury amalgams are dangerous. The ADA held patents on mercury amalgams that produced revenue and income for the ADA, and the ADA claims mercury amalgams are safe, but cannot prove it based on any type of scientific research. The basis of safety is the fact that they have been used for 170 years. In addition, the ADA claims they cannot be sued by anyone as it relates to the mercury danger. The ADA's position on mercury amalgams has created sanctioned illness in our society based on its unquestioned authority and power.

Succinctly, the ADA is a political entity, not a consumer watchdog. It has a conflict of interest and should be disbanded at least in its current state. Precedent has been set when the governor of California disbanded the California Dental Board. A totally new board was sworn in 2002. Replacing the current ADA should be a responsible organization that's sole mission is to insure materials that are placed in our mouths will not adversely affect our health.

The Hippocratic Oath is an oath of ethical professional behavior sworn to by new physicians and dentists. One of the tenants of this oath is "First Do No Harm". In other words do not complicate a problem by adding to it. This is a basic philosophy of every doctor in this country. However, based on the information that is available every dentist that inserts a mercury amalgam is causing harm. The Hippocratic Oath is being ignored. Add to the problem, if a dentist practices ethical behavior and attempts to follow an oath that is considered sacrosanct they may lose their license to practice dentistry. State regulators prevent informed consent and attempt to punish dentists who believe in educating consumers. They are precluded from discussing the controversy surrounding the mercury amalgam and the science that has created this controversy. This creates a dilemma for every dentist that wants to discontinue the usage of mercury. They cannot do it and remain in practice. Dentistry today is simply "drill, fill and bill". No questions. The ADA mafia insures this century old practice will continue.

The ADA is not changing its position and politically the ADA will continue to survive the onslaught of charges many us make on a daily basis. So how do we change the current situation? A few possibilities exist. First, as more and more consumers become aware of the toxic effects of amalgams usage the grass roots concept of change might evolve. Second, insurance companies might recognize the short term versus the long-term implications. In the short term consumers demand insurance companies pay for the removal of amalgams, but in the long term disease and illness decrease thereby creating a more profitable entity thus benefiting shareholders. Third, the government will realize the travesty that currently exists and mandate change. For instance, currently $2,000,000,000 is spent on kidney disease. The total Medicare expense due to the use of mercury amalgams is in the billions. As taxpayers that is government waste. In reality as taxpayers we are financially supporting the usage of mercury. Rather ironic.

Write your congressman, senators and the Department of Health, Education and Welfare, the National Institute of Health, the EPA and Secretary of the Treasury. All it takes is one individual with the authority to champion this cause. Make noise.

It is still possible to champion change. Don't get frustrated. Just recently the governor of Maine signed bill LD 697. This requires the installation of Dental Amalgam Separator Systems in all dental offices. This type of system will remove 98% of the mercury in wastewater discharges that results from dental work of mercury fillings. The use of these systems drastically reduces the amount of mercury that is discharged into our rivers and streams by dental offices. We are cleaning up our environment. Separators are required in other states and cities.

In addition, support the Watson Bill (#4163). This bill was introduced in April 2002 by co-sponsors Diane Watson, D-CA, and Dan Burton, R-IN. The proposed legislation bans to use of mercury amalgam in children under six and in pregnant women, and in five years bans its use in this country.

History suggests change takes place when change benefits society. This was demonstrated when the Industrial Revolution transformed our country. Recently the information and technology revolution changed everyone's productivity and altered the way business is conducted by every corporation. Health care is big business. Eventually consumers will demand health care that benefits the individual. When this occurs the health care revolution will take place. The traditional allopathic approach will be replaced by solving the reasons for disease not drugs to address the symptoms.

The concept of "First Do No Harm" cannot be challenged as one of the most important elements of healthcare. Mercury is a poison, and should not be placed in our mouth. The illness and disease that follow is a felony that is being committed by everyone involved in the perpetuation of

180

mercury amalgam usage. The assailant is aware of the crime and is committing the crime without consequences. The person paying the price for the felony is the victim not the assailant. Meanwhile, the assailant continues his crime on other unsuspecting citizens decade after decade. It is both ironic and criminal. It violates every tenant of the principal of "First Do No Harm".

__It's time to stop the disaster that has been promulgated by the Great Dental Deception during the past two centuries. It's time to ban the use of mercury in all dental procedures.__

FOR UPDATED INFORMATION VISIT

WWW. THEGREATDENTALDECEPTION.COM